IBS

This edition first published in Canada in 2007 by Whitecap Books,
351 Lynn Ave., North Vancouver, British Columbia, Canada, V7J 2C4.

www.whitecap.ca

ISBN 1 55285 878 2
ISBN 978 1 55285 878 3

Chief Executive: Juliet Rogers
Publishing Director: Kay Scarlett

Project manager: Emma Hutchinson
Editor: Kim Rowney
Design concept: Susanne Geppert
Designer: Anthony Vandenberg
Photographer: Ian Hofstetter
Stylists: Jane Collins and Katy Holder
Food preparation: Andrew DeSousa and Joanne Kelly
Recipes by: Grace Campbell, Michelle Earl and members of the Murdoch Books Test Kitchen
Production: Maiya Levitch

First published in 2007 by Murdoch Books Pty Limited.

Printed by Sing Cheong Printing Co. Ltd. in 2007. PRINTED IN HONG KONG.

The Publisher and stylists would like to thank Dinosaur Designs, Mud Australia, Bison Homewares and IKEA for
assistance in the photography of this book.

IMPORTANT: Those who might be at risk from the effects of salmonella poisoning (the elderly, pregnant women,
young children and those suffering from immune deficiency diseases) should consult their doctor with any
concerns about eating raw eggs.

CONVERSION GUIDE: You may find cooking times vary depending on the oven you are using. For fan-forced ovens,
as a general rule, set the oven temperature to 20°C (35°F) lower than indicated in the recipe. We have used 20 ml
(4 teaspoon) tablespoon measures. If you are using a 15 ml (3 teaspoon) tablespoon, for most recipes the difference
will not be noticeable. However, for recipes using baking powder, gelatine, bicarbonate of soda (baking soda), small
amounts of flour and cornflour (cornstarch), add an extra teaspoon for each tablespoon specified.

EATWELLLIVEWELL

with
IBS

High-fibre recipes and tips

Introductory text by Dr Susanna Holt (PhD, Dietitian)

whitecap

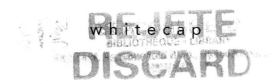

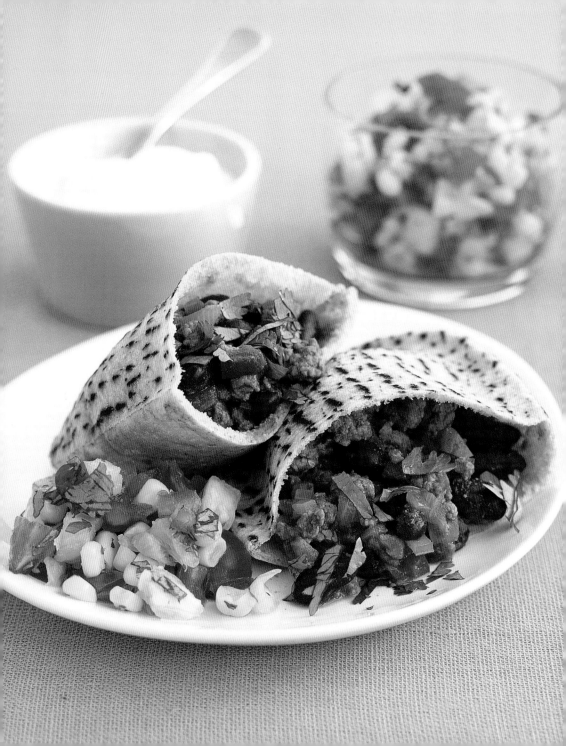

CONTENTS

GOOD HEALTH WITH HIGH FIBRE

We all know that fibre helps keep our digestive system healthy, but not everyone knows that high-fibre diets have so much more to offer. A fibre-rich diet helps control your weight, blood sugar and cholesterol levels and reduces your risk of developing heart disease, type 2 diabetes and certain cancers.

Fibre—the natural laxative

Recent studies have shown that a high intake of fibre from wholegrain cereal foods, such as natural muesli, wholegrain bread and brown rice, is associated with a lower risk of digestive tract cancers (such as mouth, stomach and bowel). Given all of fibre's healthy features, it's a shame that we don't include more of this natural laxative in our daily diets.

Oral laxatives, sold over the counter, continue to be top-selling pharmaceutical products in all modern countries around the world. In fact, laxative sales are still increasing as the proportion of elderly people in these countries continues to grow. Regular laxative use should be avoided because you may need ever-increasing doses to achieve the desired effect, which increases the risk of other health problems. Many people would not need to use laxatives if they increased their fibre and water intake and their physical activity—a simple, healthy remedy.

Are you eating enough fibre?

Health surveys continue to show that most people in industrialized countries still don't eat enough fibre on a regular basis for good long-term health. You may find this surprising after you read the following pages and learn how easy it is to add more fibre to your daily diet.

Despite ongoing health campaigns that try to educate people about the importance of a nutritious diet, dietary surveys show that many people regularly eat less than the recommended amounts of fruit, vegetables, wholegrain products and legumes. However, the good news is that simply by changing your eating habits to include more fibre-rich foods and less fat and overly processed foods in your diet, you can achieve a lot of healthy eating goals at the same time—you will increase your intake of fibre and healthy antioxidants while decreasing your intake of saturated fat. A healthier diet together with regular exercise will help make you look good and feel good, and will reduce your risk of weight gain and

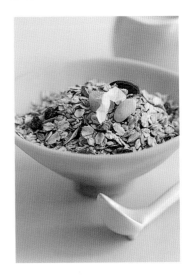

the diseases that many people develop as they get older, such as high blood pressure, high blood cholesterol, haemorrhoids and diabetes. By being well nourished and active, you'll also find it easier to perform both mental and physical tasks, which helps make them more enjoyable.

How can this book help you?

It's not hard to improve your diet and lifestyle, you just need to get organized. Schedule regular exercise into your weekly activities and keep your refrigerator and pantry well stocked with healthy foods. This book will also help you: it provides information about the health powers of a fibre-rich diet and practical advice about how you can easily increase your fibre intake. It contains a variety of tested recipes that provide good amounts of fibre while meeting other healthy eating guidelines too, such as being lower in fat. Most of the recipes in this book provide at least 5–6 grams of fibre per serve. However, a few of the baking recipes contain less than 5 grams of fibre per serve, but they provide more fibre than the regular version of the recipe. Among the recipes, you'll find options for healthy, everyday meals that the whole family will enjoy, as well as dishes that can be prepared for special occasions.

It's never too late to start roughing it. Increase your fibre intake and reap the health benefits of a high-fibre diet based on fruits, vegetables, legumes and grain products.

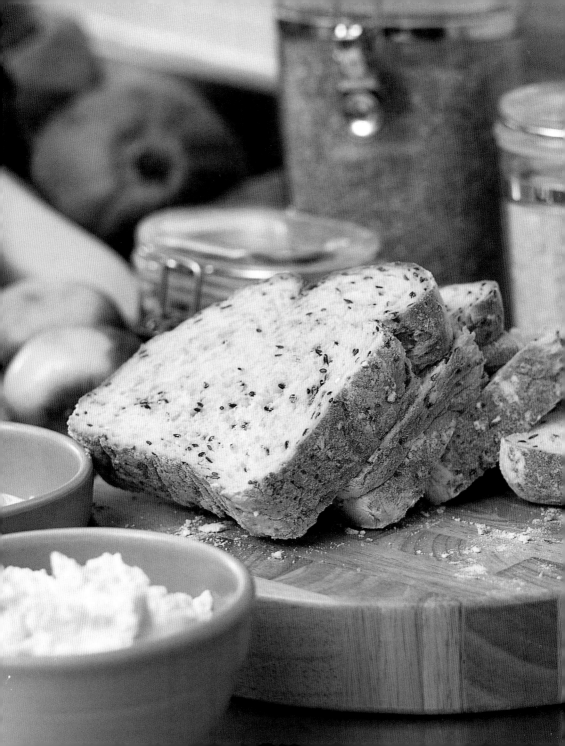

What is fibre?

Dietary fibre, also known as roughage, is found in plant foods, such as grains, nuts, seeds, legumes, fruit, vegetables and seaweed. Animal foods, such as meat, fish, chicken, eggs and cow's milk, do not contain any fibre.

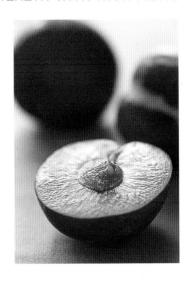

Fibre refers to any component of plant foods that cannot be digested (broken down) by human digestive enzymes. The fibrous strings in celery and green beans, and the white pithy membrane of citrus fruit are visible examples of fibre. Other than lignin, the different types of fibre are all types of carbohydrate because they are made up of chains of individual sugar units bound together. However, unlike the other dietary carbohydrates (sugars and starches), the sugar chains in fibre cannot be broken down by our digestive enzymes. So, fibre remains undigested as it passes through our stomach and small intestine and moves down to the lower intestine.

Different types of fibre

There are two main types of dietary fibre: insoluble and soluble fibre. Plant foods typically contain a mixture of these two types of fibre. There are also two other types of compounds in plant foods—resistant starch and non-digestible oligosaccharides—that scientists classify as fibre, because they are indigestible carbohydrates that have fibre-like effects in our body.

Different types of dietary fibre have different effects in our body due to differences in their chemical structure.

Insoluble fibre: includes cellulose, hemicellulose and lignin, which make up the structural parts of plant cell walls. Insoluble fibre doesn't dissolve in water but it can soak up a lot of water inside our stomach and intestines. The indigestible fibre and extra water increases the bulk of the food contents, which helps push the digested food matter through our digestive system, removing waste materials and preventing constipation. You can think of insoluble fibre as a natural laxative that, together with water, helps flush out our system. Good sources of insoluble fibre include wholegrain bread, brown rice, wheat bran, rice bran, nuts, seeds, legumes and unpeeled fruit and vegetables.

Soluble fibre: includes pectins, gums and mucilage, which are mainly found around and inside plant cells. Soluble fibre absorbs water or partially dissolves in water and forms a gel-like substance in the stomach and intestines. This can help slow down the rate of food digestion and reduce the extent to which your blood sugar level rises as you digest a meal (if enough soluble fibre is consumed in the meal). Like insoluble fibre, the water absorbed by soluble fibre also adds bulk to food contents and helps push them through our digestive system. However, soluble fibre differs from insoluble fibre in that it can be fermented by the 'friendly' bacteria that naturally live in our large intestine. This process benefits both us and our bacteria. The fatty acids that are produced during the fermentation of soluble fibre provide the bacteria with a source of energy and also produce some beneficial effects in our body, such as helping to reduce our risk of heart disease and bowel cancer.

Good sources of soluble fibre include oat bran, psyllium fibre, linseeds (flax seeds), barley and legumes, such as chickpeas and cannellini beans. Due to their gelling effects, soluble fibres are added to certain processed foods, such as jams and sauces, as thickening or setting agents (for example, pectin and gums).

Resistant starch: is starch (a type of carbohydrate) that is not digested in the small intestine and passes into the large intestine where it can be fermented by bacteria. Resistant starch does not increase the bulk of food matter in our gut like soluble and insoluble fibre because it doesn't absorb lots of water. However, like soluble fibre, it can be fermented by the bacteria that live in our large intestine, which is how we derive health benefits from this nutrient.

Some resistant starch cannot be digested because it is physically trapped inside foods where our digestive enzymes can't reach it, such as inside seeds, lentils and whole grains. Some resistant starch is formed in starchy foods after they have been cooked and cooled. For example, in bread, cornflakes, cold cooked potatoes (cold potato salad), rice (sushi) and pasta (pasta salad). Recently, some food manufacturers have started adding resistant starch (such as Hi-maize) to processed foods, such as white bread, snack bars and breakfast cereals, to increase their 'fibre' content.

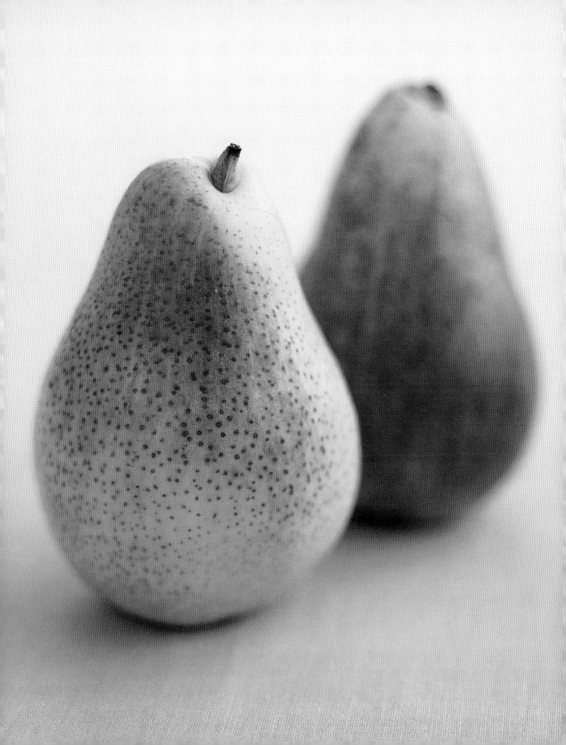

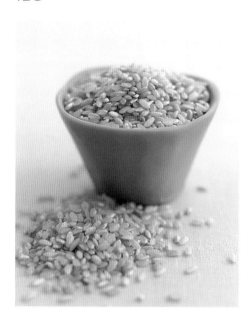

Non-digestible oligosaccharides: are small carbohydrates (bigger than a sugar but smaller than a starch) that cannot be digested by enzymes in the human stomach and small intestine. Like soluble fibre and resistant starch, they pass undigested into the large intestine where they are fermented by bacteria, resulting in the production of gas and fatty acids. This is one reason why some people complain of gas after they eat a meal of baked beans. Oligosaccharides include raffinose, inulin, stachyose and oligofructose, and they are found in legumes and certain vegetables (such as artichokes, leeks, onions and garlic). Inulin is added to some processed foods, such as some brands of yoghurt, as a prebiotic to help stimulate the growth of beneficial bacteria living in our lower intestine.

How does fibre help keep my digestive system healthy?

The human digestive system is a very efficient system that we take for granted until something goes wrong. Many people in industrialized countries eat a low-fibre diet and develop gastrointestinal problems as they age, such as chronic constipation, haemorrhoids, varicose veins, diverticular disease and colon (bowel) cancer. It generally takes 2 to 36 hours for food to be digested and pass through the body, depending on the type of food you've eaten, your fluid intake and any other health conditions you may have. A high-fibre diet helps speed up the process of food elimination, and is an easy way you can protect your digestive system from future problems.

After we eat a meal, insoluble and soluble fibre in the food absorbs and binds a lot of water and as a result the food matter becomes larger, softer and bulkier. The increased bulk stimulates the process of peristalsis, where muscular contractions push the digested food down towards the lower (large) intestine. This process occurs more quickly and easily with a high-fibre diet. Low-fibre meals soak up less water in our gastrointestinal tract, so low-fibre food waste is smaller, harder and takes longer to move through the digestive system, and are more difficult to pass from the body. (The slowing down effect of soluble fibre on food digestion tends to be overridden by the bulking effect of insoluble fibre, unless a large amount of soluble fibre is eaten. Most meals contain more insoluble fibre than soluble fibre.)

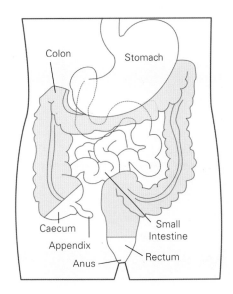

Small intestine and large intestine/colon (shaded)

Constipation—what an irritation!

Constipation is defined as having fewer than three bowel movements a week. However, some people will feel constipated if they don't have at least one bowel movement a day (normal stool elimination can vary between people from three times a day to three times a week). Constipation typically occurs when the muscular contractions of the large intestine are slow or sluggish, causing the stool to move too slowly. As a result, the stool becomes hard and dry and more difficult to eliminate. Constipation is a common problem in industrialized societies (no wonder so many people take something to read when they go to the toilet). Constipation is particularly common among older people and is typically caused by a low-fibre diet, a lack of physical activity, dehydration, certain medications or health problems (including the overuse of laxatives).

You can prevent or treat constipation by increasing your fibre (20–35 grams a day) and water intake and by increasing your physical activity. It's important to avoid chronic constipation because it can lead to complications, such as haemorrhoids, anal tears or a rectal prolapse due to the increased strain required for bowel movements. See your doctor for advice if you regularly suffer from constipation. You could also see a dietitian for advice about how you can gradually increase your fibre intake.

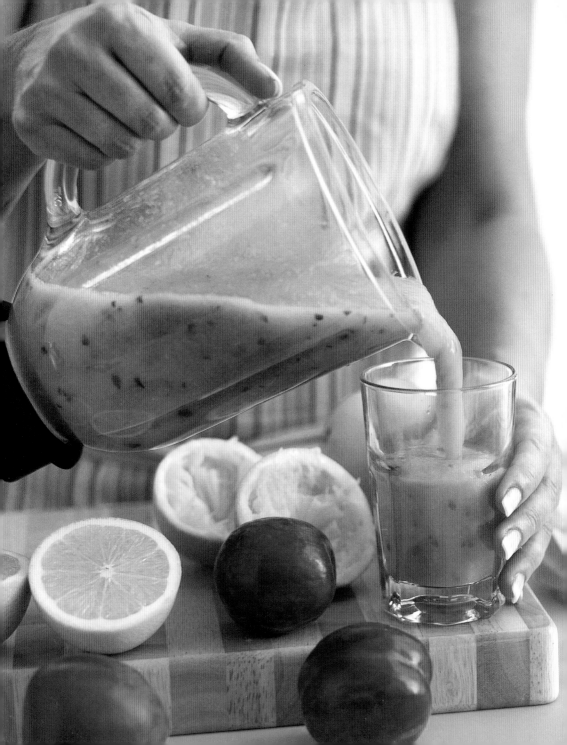

Diverticular disease

After the age of 40, many people develop diverticula, which are small pouches that bulge out of the inner part of the colon (like an inner tube that pokes out of a weak spot in a bicycle tyre). This condition is called diverticulosis or diverticular disease. If one or more of these pouches becomes inflamed or infected, the condition is called diverticulitis, which affects 10–25% of people with diverticula. Many people with diverticular disease do not have any discomfort, but others experience cramps, abdominal bloating and constipation. Stress, medications and other health disorders, such as irritable bowel syndrome, can cause similar symptoms, so it's important to see your doctor if you regularly experience these symptoms.

Health benefits of a high-fibre diet
- Prevents constipation, haemorrhoids and diverticular disease
- Increases the number of 'friendly' bacteria in the colon
- Lowers the risk of colon cancer
- Makes weight control easier
- Helps control your blood sugar level and blood cholesterol level
- Reduces the risk of type 2 diabetes and heart disease

Diverticular disease can lead to complications such as infections, tears or a blockage that requires surgery. The most common cause of diverticular disease is thought to be constipation resulting from a low-fibre, high-fat diet. Constipation makes it much harder for a person to pass a stool, and the increased pressure could cause weak spots in the colon to bulge out and form diverticula. Diverticular disease and constipation are rare among rural communities in less-developed countries where people are very active and eat high-fibre diets. A high-fibre diet with plenty of water is the only treatment required by most people with diverticulosis. In some cases, a doctor may recommend a fibre supplement mixed with water.

Irritable bowel syndrome

Irritable bowel syndrome (IBS) is a functional bowel disorder, which does not appear to be due to any physical abnormalities, and is characterized by abdominal pain, gas, bloating and cramps with constipation and/or diarrhoea. IBS is not a well-researched condition, and no clear cause of IBS has been established. However, possible causes include certain dietary factors and problems with the bowel's muscular contractions due to illness, infection or psychological factors such as prolonged stress. If you have had abdominal pain plus diarrhoea and/or constipation, on and off for at least 12 weeks in the last year, then see your doctor for an assessment. These symptoms could be due to IBS or another condition, such as lactose intolerance or coeliac disease. It's important to get a proper diagnosis, so you can get the proper treatment.

There are a number of dietary changes a person with IBS can make to reduce pain, discomfort and bowel problems. In particular, it can be helpful to avoid or reduce the intake of spicy foods, oily/fatty and fried foods, dairy foods (even when there is no lactose intolerance), chocolate, coffee (regular and decaffeinated), alcohol and carbonated beverages. The following things can help reduce IBS symptoms, but there is a lot of individual variation (some things work better for some people): eat foods with soluble fibre, substitute dairy products with non-dairy versions, and eat small regular meals (for example, six small meals instead of three big ones). Some people also find that they can't eat large quantities of foods rich in insoluble fibre, such as bran cereals, legumes or unpeeled vegetables. Other people find that fibre-rich foods can help alleviate constipation, but may not help people who suffer from diarrhoea or abdominal cramping.

People with IBS need individually tailored medical and dietary advice provided by a doctor and an experienced dietitian. The advice needs to suit the individual's specific problems, and can vary at times depending on whether constipation or diarrhoea is the predominant problem. Doctors usually recommend that people with IBS eat enough fibre to enable them to have soft, painless bowel movements. Medication may be required to alleviate cramping and pain.

Colon (bowel) cancer

The colon is another name for the large intestine, which makes up the second half of our digestive tract. After we eat a meal, our gall bladder squirts bile acids into our small intestine to help with the digestion and absorption of dietary fat. Most of these bile acids are absorbed back into the body and recycled, but some bile acids bind to the fibre in the food matter and move down to the large intestine. Bacteria in the large intestine then metabolize these bile acids into secondary bile acids, which have been shown to have a carcinogenic or cancer-promoting effect on the cells of the colon. Epidemiological research studies have shown that low-fibre, high-fat diets lead to elevated faecal concentrations of secondary bile acids, which is associated with an increased risk of colon cancer.

A low-fat, high-fibre diet may be particularly helpful for preventing colon cancer in people who have an increased risk of developing the condition. A recent American research study has shown that a low-fat diet plus a daily supplement of wheat bran reduced the size and the number of colonic polyps in patients with a history of recurring polyps. Colonic polyps are abnormal tissue growths that occur in the mucous membrane of the colon, which increase the risk of colon cancer. They can be flat or raised on a stalk, and some can be removed surgically. Most polyps don't cause any symptoms, so they are usually only discovered when doctors perform routine colon cancer screening tests (such as a rectal examination or a colonoscopy).

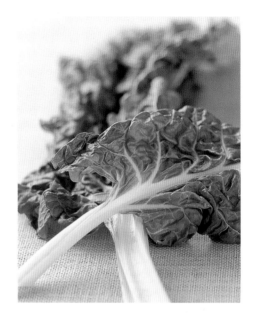

A high-fibre diet with a relatively low fat content is thought to reduce our risk of developing colon cancer in several ways. Firstly, high-fibre meals speed up the movement of food matter through the colon, which reduces the amount of time our colon is in contact with any cancer-promoting chemicals in the faecal contents, such as secondary bile acids. Fibre also increases the water content and bulk of the faecal matter, effectively diluting any carcinogenic compounds. Secondly, soluble fibre, non-digestible oligosaccharides and resistant starch can be fermented by bacteria in the colon, resulting in the production of gas and short-chain fatty acids. These fatty acids have a number of beneficial effects: they are used by the bacteria as an energy source and are also absorbed into our bloodstream through the wall of the colon. They make the colon more acidic, which helps protect the colon's lining from cancerous changes (polyp formation) and increases the absorption of minerals. They also stimulate the production of immune cells and improve the barrier properties of the colon wall (inhibiting inflammation and the adhesion of irritants). By providing energy, the fatty acids also enable the bacteria to divide and grow in numbers, increasing the number of friendly bacteria in your colon. Reducing your intake of fat and processed foods and increasing your fibre intake are simple things you can do to reduce your risk of developing colon cancer.

Good sources of fibre

Food	Serve size	Approximate fibre content of serve (grams)
Processed wheat bran cereal (All-Bran)	¾ cup	15.1 g
Natural untoasted muesli (average)	⅔ cup	8.9 g
Bran flakes	1 cup	6.5 g
Oat bran, unprocessed	1 tbsp	1.8 g
Wheat bran, unprocessed	1 tbsp	2.2 g
Wholegrain bread, regular, supermarket variety	2 slices	3.3 g
Pumpernickel bread	1 slice	4.2 g
Brown rice, boiled or steamed	1 cup	2.7 g
Wholemeal (whole-wheat) pasta, boiled	1 cup	8.4 g
Barley, boiled	½ cup	3.3 g
Baked beans, tinned	¾ cup	9.9 g
Chickpeas, tinned, drained	½ cup	4.1 g
Kidney beans, tinned, drained	½ cup	6.2 g
Figs, dried	3 figs	8.1 g
Apricots, dried	8 halves	2.6 g
Strawberries, raw	½ cup halves	1.8 g
Apple, raw, unpeeled	1 medium	3.3 g
Pear, green, raw, unpeeled	1 medium	3.7 g
Orange, raw, peeled	1 medium	2.6 g
Nectarine, raw, unpeeled	1 medium	3.6 g
Sauerkraut, tinned	½ cup	2.1 g
Broccoli, cooked	1 cup	4.2 g
Corn, cooked	1 medium cob	2.4 g
Green beans, cooked	½ cup	2.0 g
Spinach, cooked	½ cup chopped	4.6 g
Peas, green, cooked	½ cup	4.6 g
Brussels sprouts, cooked	4 sprouts	2.9 g
Potato, cooked whole, with skin	1 medium	2.8 g
Almonds, raw	⅓ cup	4.4 g
Pistachios, raw	⅓ cup	3.7 g
Peanuts, raw	⅓ cup	4.2 g
Sunflower seeds or pepitas (pumpkin seeds)	1 tbsp	1.4 g

A healthy lower fat diet, based on a variety of plant foods, provides fibre as well as plenty of other healthy nutrients, such as vitamins, minerals, antioxidants and phytochemicals. Fibre alone isn't responsible for all of the health benefits you get from a healthy fibre-rich diet. Choosing wholegrain cereal products with visible fibre instead of 'white' refined versions is an easy way to increase your intake of fibre and other healthy nutrients. Choosing wholegrain foods with a low glycaemic index (GI) value is particularly beneficial (for example, wholegrain bread instead of white bread; natural muesli instead of cornflakes; brown basmati rice instead of white) because they are digested and absorbed at a relatively slow rate, which prevents a large rise and fall in your blood sugar level. The smaller rise in your blood sugar level means that your body needs less insulin (a hormone) to absorb the sugar from the bloodstream. A lower insulin diet is thought to help reduce the risk of developing colon cancer. An easy way to lower the insulin-raising effect of your diet is to choose low-GI carbohydrate-rich foods as part of a healthy lower fat diet based on grains, legumes, fruit and vegetables. Not only does this kind of diet help reduce your risk of colon cancer, but it also makes weight control easier and lowers the risk of diabetes, heart disease and other cancers too.

Healthy eating and lifestyle guidelines
- Eat a variety of nutritious foods each day.
- Base your diet on vegetables, fruit, legumes and grain products (mostly wholegrain and low-GI).
- Eat a variety of different coloured fruits and vegetables each week.
- Eat a lower fat diet with a low saturated fat content.
- Drink alcohol in moderation, if at all.
- Limit your intake of salt and added sugars.
- Regularly eat foods that contain iron and calcium.
- Maintain a healthy weight and be physically active.
- Drink plenty of water each day.

How does fibre help with weight control?

Many research studies have found that overweight people easily lose weight when their diet is modified to include more healthy foods with less fat and more fibre. Think how easy it is to drink a glass of apple juice, but how difficult it would be to eat three whole apples in the same amount of time. Although you're consuming roughly the same amount of kilojoules, the whole apples are going to make you full much faster than the juice, simply because your jaws have to work much harder to chew and swallow the larger volume of whole apples. This slows down your rate of eating and gives your brain time to register the growing feeling of fullness in your stomach.

Tips for increasing your fibre intake

- Choose wholegrain bread instead of white or wholemeal (whole-wheat).
- Choose brown rice and pasta instead of white.
- Serve main meals with salads and plenty of vegetables.
- Eat whole fruit rather than drinking fruit juice.
- Have fruit-based desserts.
- Snack on dried fruit, fresh fruit, fresh vegetable sticks, nuts and seeds.
- Add boiled or tinned drained legumes to salads, soups, stews and curries.
- Choose a high-fibre breakfast cereal (natural muesli, bran-based cereals, psyllium-enriched flakes) and serve with fresh or dried fruit.
- Add some seeds or nuts to fruit salad, yoghurt, fruit crumbles and baking recipes.
- Make porridge from traditional wholegrain oats rather than quick-cooking or instant oats.
- Use wholemeal (whole-wheat) flour or stoneground flour in baking recipes.
- Eat more vegetarian meals and stir-fries with lots of vegetables.
- Include lots of salad vegetables or tabouleh in your sandwiches and bread rolls.
- Explore your local health food shop to find high-fibre breakfast cereals, breads and snacks.
- Serve a variety of salads (bean salads, tabouleh) and different grainy breads at barbecues and picnics. Spray vegetables with olive oil and add them to a barbecue.
- When you serve rice, add some lentils or barley for extra fibre, nutrients and flavour. This will also lower the GI of the rice.
- If you want second helpings at dinner, make sure it's mostly vegetables.
- Add coarsely grated vegetables to cakes and muffins; and add more vegetables to pasta sauces, soups, stews and stir-fries.
- Take your own lunch to work: minestrone soup; salad; grainy bread rolls.
- Add vegetables to your breakfast, by adding them to omelettes or serving eggs with mushrooms, asparagus, tomatoes, spinach and wholegrain toast.

You may not even be able to eat three apples in one go, but you could easily drink them in a glass of juice. Unlike the whole apples that still contain their fibre intact, the fibre in the apple juice has been 'ground up' into smaller particles by the juicing process. The ground-up fibre will be less effective in your body, because it will be less able to bind water and increase the bulk of your stomach contents.

Just like the apples, cereal grains such as wheat become easier to eat and less filling as you progressively grind them up from whole grains into cracked grains, then into coarse and fine flour. They also become more easily digested, which increases the blood sugar and insulin effect they produce. Bread made from fine wheat flour has a higher blood sugar effect (GI value) than bread made from coarsely ground flour or bread with whole grains in it. Consequently, the fibre content on a food label may not always be a good indication of how 'healthy' that fibre is. Some brands of wholemeal (whole-wheat) bread have a similar fibre content to some grainy breads, but the fibre is more ground up and not as effective as the fibre in the wholegrain bread. Similarly, some types of wholegrain bread have more fibre in them than other varieties. Look for wholegrain bread with lots of visible grains in it. The more grains, the more intact fibre.

Plant foods are more filling and useful for weight control when they are less processed and closer to their natural state (for example, brown rice instead of white rice, wholegrain bread instead of white or wholemeal/whole-wheat bread). Foods with intact or less-processed fibre that are more difficult to chew and swallow will help slow

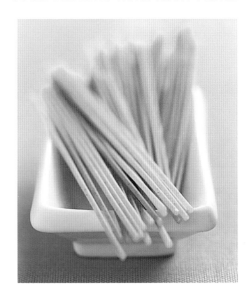

down your eating rate and make it easier for you to realize when you're starting to feel full. The nerves and muscles that are activated while you chew and swallow foods send signals to your brain to stimulate the sensation of fullness. Choosing foods that are harder to chew and swallow can make it harder for you to overeat, making weight control easier. It's possible to eat filling, satisfying meals and still keep your weight in check. Similarly, you don't need to starve yourself to lose weight, you just need to make smarter food choices focusing on both the type and amount of food you eat. Eat unpeeled fruit and vegetables, and choose brown rice and wholegrain bread. Don't mash your potatoes, eat them whole in their skin as baked potatoes. Eat fruit instead of drinking it, and boil legumes instead of using tinned ones that are softer.

How can fibre reduce the risk of diabetes?

A high-fibre diet can help reduce your risk of developing type 2 diabetes or help you control your blood sugar level if you have the condition. Soluble fibre in food can form a viscous gel when mixed with fluid in the digestive tract, which makes it harder for digestive enzymes to reach the food particles. This slows down the rate of carbohydrate digestion, which results in a slower, more steady release of sugar (glucose) into your bloodstream after a meal.

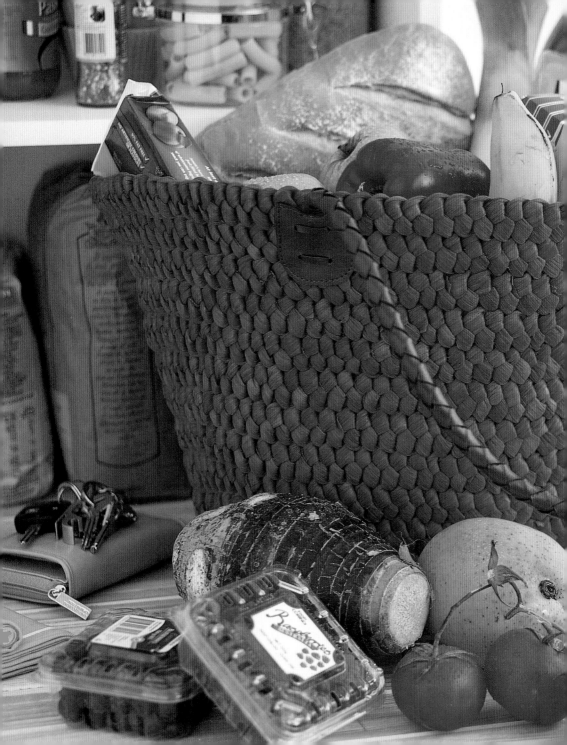

A lower fat, high-fibre diet based on plant foods plus regular exercise reduces the risk of developing type 2 diabetes as you get older. Further protection can be obtained if you mostly eat low-GI carbohydrate-containing foods and healthier sources of dietary fat (monounsaturated and omega-3 polyunsaturated fats). A healthy diet and active lifestyle make your body's tissues more sensitive to the effects of insulin, so you need to produce less insulin in order for your body to process the foods you eat. In contrast, a high-fat, high-GI, low-fibre diet requires more insulin to be metabolized, which increases the risk of weight gain, insulin resistance and type 2 diabetes.

How does fibre reduce the risk of heart disease?

Powerful evidence that a high-fibre diet reduces the risk of heart disease comes from several large research studies, including one that has been tracking the dietary habits and health problems of 43,757 men over a long period of time. Men who ate more than 25 grams of fibre per day had a 36% lower risk of developing heart disease than those who consumed less than 15 grams of fibre per day. The protective effect is not due to fibre alone. The lower intake of fat and the higher intake of vitamins, minerals, antioxidants and phytochemicals that occurs when people eat more fruit, vegetables and wholegrain products also produce the health benefits.

For people who find it difficult to eat a lot of fibre-rich foods, a low-fat diet and a soluble fibre supplement can be used to 'treat' a high blood cholesterol level and help reduce the risk of heart disease. Research studies have shown that a daily soluble fibre supplement (10–30 grams psyllium fibre, 6–40 grams pectin, 8–36 grams guar gum, 25–100 grams oat bran or barley bran, 100–150 grams dried legumes) can reduce the level of 'bad' LDL (low-density lipoprotein) cholesterol in the blood by as much as 5–10%. Similarly, eating two serves of oats per day can lower blood cholesterol by 2–3% within a few months, even without any other dietary changes. This effect is thought to be due to soluble fibre binding to dietary cholesterol and bile acids in the digestive tract and being excreted with the faeces rather than being absorbed by the body. This means the liver will need to use some cholesterol from the bloodstream to make new bile acids to replace those that have been lost. There is also some scientific evidence that suggests that the short-chain fatty acids produced by the bacterial fermentation of fibre can slow down the rate of cholesterol production in the liver. (Note: fibre supplements have not been shown to be effective for weight loss. You need to eat less fat and more fibre-rich foods for weight control.)

23

How much fibre should I be eating?

In Australia and New Zealand, health authorities currently recommend that healthy adult males eat 38 grams of fibre per day and females eat 28 grams per day, from a variety of foods. Other countries have similar targets, so a general target to aim for is 25–30 grams per day. Dietary surveys indicate that most people eat less than 20 grams per day due to low intakes of fruit, vegetables, wholegrain products and legumes. Due to their smaller size and appetites, children need less fibre than adults. As a general guide, the daily fibre target for children aged 3–18 years is their age plus 5 grams of fibre per day (for example, a 9-year-old child needs at least 9 + 5 = 14 grams of fibre per day).

What's the best way to increase my fibre intake?

Eating more fibre is an easy thing to do because fibre is found in so many foods. The other good news is that you don't need to worry about other nutritional goals at the same time. There is one general healthy eating plan that reduces the risk of all common nutrition-related illnesses that affect so many people as they get older—weight gain, high blood pressure, high blood cholesterol, heart disease, type 2 diabetes and certain cancers. All you need to do is follow the general healthy eating guidelines recommended by health authorities (for healthy people over 2 years of age), and make your diet more natural by eating mostly fruit, vegetables, grain foods

The balanced high-fibre diet pyramid

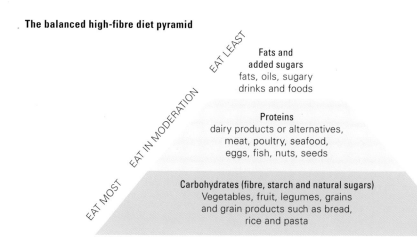

EAT LEAST

Fats and
added sugars
fats, oils, sugary
drinks and foods

EAT IN MODERATION

Proteins
dairy products or alternatives,
meat, poultry, seafood,
eggs, fish, nuts, seeds

EAT MOST

Carbohydrates (fibre, starch and natural sugars)
Vegetables, fruit, legumes, grains
and grain products such as bread,
rice and pasta

and legumes. This means that most of the food you eat each day should come from these four food groups. You can then add moderate amounts of lower fat protein-rich foods (lower fat dairy products or alternatives, eggs, lean meat and poultry, fish, seafood) and small amounts of fat (oils, margarine, avocados, olives, sauces, seeds, nuts and dressings). This will increase your intake of fibre, antioxidants and phytochemicals while decreasing your intake of saturated fat, salt and added sugars. It's recommended that you eat moderate amounts of lower fat protein-rich foods. See a dietitian if you need help working out the types and amounts of foods you should be eating

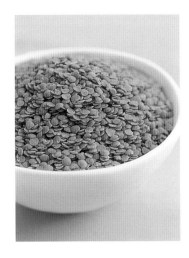

each day. In general, each day you should aim to eat: 5 serves of vegetables (including legumes); 3–4 serves of fruit; and 4 serves of grain-based foods. Try to eat at least 2 serves of legumes in your diet each week.

- 1 serve of vegetables = 1 cup of fresh salad or ½ cup of cooked vegetables.
- 1 serve of fruit = 1 medium-sized piece of fruit; 2 small-sized pieces; 1 cup of fresh fruit pieces; ½ cup of fruit juice; or 1½ tablespoons of dried fruit.
- 1 serve of legumes = ½ cup of cooked legumes.
- 1 serve of grain-based food = 2 slices of bread or 1 medium bread roll; 1 cup of cooked rice, pasta or noodles; 1 cup of cooked porridge or 1⅓ cups of breakfast cereal or ½ cup of natural muesli.

Changing over to a high-fibre diet

If your fibre intake has previously been low, then it's best to increase your fibre and water intake gradually. This will give your digestive system time to adapt and help you avoid any uncomfortable abdominal problems, such as bloating and excess gas, that can occur if you suddenly start eating high-fibre meals. If you and your family normally eat white bread, then start by switching to a wholegrain bread that's not too dense. After a while, you can start buying even grainier breads. There are plenty of delicious grainy breads with different seeds and grains in them that will appeal to different family members. It's very important to include high-fibre foods in children's diets,

Comparison of fibre content in a low-fibre and high-fibre diet over one day

Low fibre	(grams fibre)	High fibre	(grams fibre)
Breakfast			
Puffed rice cereal	0.7	Natural muesli	6.4
Reduced-fat milk	0.0	Reduced-fat milk	0.0
White sugar	0.0	Unpeeled nectarine	3.1
		1 tbsp sunflower seeds	1.2
Morning snack			
Apple juice	0.5	Water	0.0
Blueberry muffin	1.3	Whole apple, including skin	3.2
Lunch			
Ham and tomato sandwich (white bread)	2.3	Ham and salad sandwich (grainy bread)	4.5
Flavoured milk	0.0	Whole orange	2.6
Dinner			
White rice	1.0	Brown rice	2.9
Beef and vegetable stir-fry	1.5	Beef and vegetable stir-fry (with more vegetables)	2.5
Dessert			
Small serve tinned fruit	1.7	Fresh fruit salad	5.9
Ice cream	0.0	Ice cream	0.0
Total fibre intake	**9.0**		**32.3**

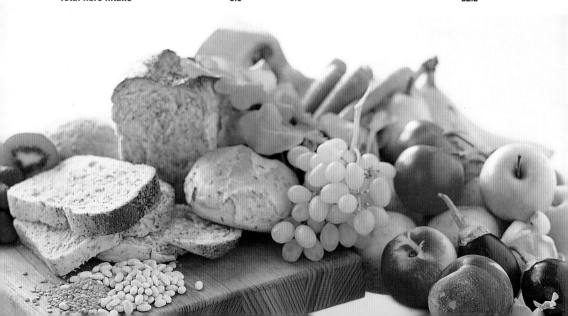

because the extra chewing helps their teeth and jaws develop properly, and also teaches them to appreciate more nutritious foods. Children who are brought up on soft white bread and soft peeled fruits often find it difficult to eat grainy bread and unpeeled fruit as they get older, so they will miss out on the health benefits these foods have to offer.

Choosing higher fibre breakfast cereals is another good way to increase your family's fibre intake. A research study showed that university students felt less hungry and more alert during the morning if they started their day with a high-fibre breakfast (such as processed bran cereal, low-fat milk, banana, wholegrain toast and jam) rather than a high-fat meal (croissant or bacon and eggs with white toast). High-fibre foods that are digested slowly, such as bran cereal, natural muesli or wholegrain porridge, provide a steady release of glucose sugar into the bloodstream, which is good for sustaining both mental and physical performance. You may find that you'll easily lose a little weight after you start increasing your fibre intake, because you may no longer need a mid-morning or afternoon snack when your main meals are higher in fibre and more filling. If you find it hard to eat a whole bowl of bran or natural muesli, then try eating half a bowl and top it with another cereal and some fresh fruit.

How to use this book

The recipes in this book have all been selected because they contain good amounts of fibre and meet other healthy eating guidelines. The nutrient content for an average serve is listed for each recipe. This is an estimate only, and can vary depending on the brand of ingredients used and due to variation in the nutrient content of natural produce. If the weight or amount of an ingredient is not specified, average or medium weights were used in the nutritional analysis. The nutritional analysis of recipes does not include any serving suggestions or garnishes, unless listed in specific quantities.

Disclaimer

This book provides general information about healthy eating based on valid information at the time of printing. It is not intended to replace any advice given to you by a qualified doctor or other mainstream health professional. It is particularly important that you consult with your doctor before making any changes to your dietary and exercise habits, if you have health problems and/or if you are taking prescription medication. Neither the author nor the publishers can be held responsible for claims arising from the inappropriate use or incorrect interpretation of any of the dietary advice described in this book.

BREAKFAST

FULL-OF-FIBRE MUESLI

MADE WITH WHOLEGRAIN OATS, NUTS, SEEDS AND DRIED FRUIT, ALL GOOD
SOURCES OF FIBRE, THIS MUESLI WILL HELP SUSTAIN YOUR ENERGY LEVELS
THROUGHOUT THE MORNING.

30 g (1 oz/⅓ cup) flaked almonds

200 g (7 oz/2 cups) wholegrain rolled
  (porridge) oats

60 g (2¼ oz/1 cup) processed bran cereal

35 g (1¼ oz/⅓ cup) wholegrain rolled
  barley

30 g (1 oz/¼ cup) pepitas (pumpkin
  seeds)

2 tbsp sunflower seeds

1 tbsp linseeds (flax seeds)

90 g (3¼ oz/¾ cup) sultanas (golden
  raisins)

185 g (6¼ oz/1 cup) chopped dried apricots

90 g (3¼ oz/½ cup) chopped dried pears

skim milk, to serve

low-fat yoghurt, to serve

PREP TIME: 15 MINUTES

COOKING TIME: 5 MINUTES

SERVES 6

Preheat the oven to 160°C (315°F/Gas 2–3). Put the almonds on a baking tray in a single layer and toast in the oven for 5 minutes, or until golden. Remove and set aside.

Put the rolled oats, processed bran cereal, rolled barley, pepitas, sunflower seeds and linseeds in a bowl, then stir to combine. Add the sultanas, apricots and pears to the bowl, then stir in the toasted almonds.

Serve with skim milk and top with some yoghurt. Add some chopped fresh fruit for extra fibre, if desired. Store any remaining muesli in an airtight container for up to 2 weeks.

nutrition per serve: Energy 1761 kJ (421 Cal); Fat 11.4 g; Saturated fat 1.4 g; Protein 10.8 g; Carbohydrate 64 g; Fibre 12.8 g; Cholesterol 0 mg

SWISS MUESLI

RUNNING OUT OF TIME IN THE MORNING IS NO EXCUSE FOR MISSING OUT ON THE BENEFITS OF A HEALTHY BREAKFAST. THIS MUESLI CAN BE PREPARED THE NIGHT BEFORE AND THEN ENJOYED THE NEXT MORNING.

100 g (3½ oz/1 cup) wholegrain rolled (porridge) oats
1 tbsp wheat germ
2 tbsp sultanas (golden raisins)
1 tbsp pepitas (pumpkin seeds)
2 tbsp chopped raw almonds or hazelnuts
125 ml (4 fl oz/½ cup) unsweetened apple juice

70 g (2½ oz/½ cup) unpeeled grated apple (1 small apple)
125 g (4½ oz/½ cup) low-fat plain yoghurt
strawberries or blueberries, to serve

PREP TIME: 10 MINUTES + 1 HOUR REFRIGERATION
COOKING TIME: NIL
SERVES 2

Combine the oats, wheat germ, sultanas, pepitas and nuts in a bowl. Pour over the apple juice and stir to combine. Cover and refrigerate for 1 hour for the oat mixture to absorb the juice, or refrigerate overnight.

Just before serving, add the grated apple and yoghurt and stir to combine. The mixture should be fairly wet but not runny. Add more or less yoghurt to achieve the desired consistency. Serve topped with fresh berries.

HINTS:
• This muesli is delicious served with other fresh fruit such as pears, peaches, plums, nectarines or apricots. Use unpeeled fruit for more fibre.
• Experiment with different ingredients to vary the flavour of the muesli. Try adding linseeds (flax seeds) or LSA (a coarsely ground mixture of linseeds, sunflower seeds and almonds) to the oat mixture. LSA can be bought ready-made from large supermarkets and health food shops.

nutrition per serve: Energy 1791 kJ (428 Cal); Fat 14 g; Saturated fat 1.7 g; Protein 14.2 g; Carbohydrate 57.7 g; Fibre 6.9 g; Cholesterol 3 mg

MULTIGRAIN PORRIDGE

**400 g (14 oz/4 cups) wholegrain rolled
  (porridge) oats**
100 g (3½ oz/1 cup) rice flakes
130 g (4½ oz/1 cup) barley flakes
130 g (4½ oz/1 cup) rye flakes
200 g (7 oz/1 cup) millet
2 tbsp sesame seeds, lightly toasted
2 tsp linseeds (flax seeds)
low-fat milk or plain yoghurt, to serve
soft brown sugar, to serve

PREP TIME: 10 MINUTES + 10 MINUTES
  SOAKING
COOKING TIME: 20 MINUTES
MAKES 16 SERVES

Put the rolled oats, rice flakes, barley flakes, rye flakes, millet, sesame seeds and linseeds in a large bowl and stir well. Store in a sealed container until ready to use.

To prepare the porridge for four people, put 250 g (9 oz/2 cups) of the dry mixture, a pinch of salt and 500 ml (17 fl oz/2 cups) water in a saucepan. Stir well, then set aside for 10 minutes (this creates a smoother, creamier porridge). Stir again and then add another 500 ml (17 fl oz/2 cups) water.

Bring to the boil over medium heat, stirring occasionally. Reduce the heat to low and simmer the porridge, stirring frequently, for 12–15 minutes, or until the mixture is soft and creamy and the grains are cooked. Serve with milk or yoghurt and brown sugar.

HINTS:
• If you like, add 60 g (2¼ oz/½ cup) sultanas (golden raisins) or a mixture of dried fruits to the dry mixture, and cook as above.
• If you prefer a creamier porridge, substitute half the water for low-fat milk.
• Look for the cereal grains and flakes in the health food aisle of your supermarket, or visit your local health food shop.

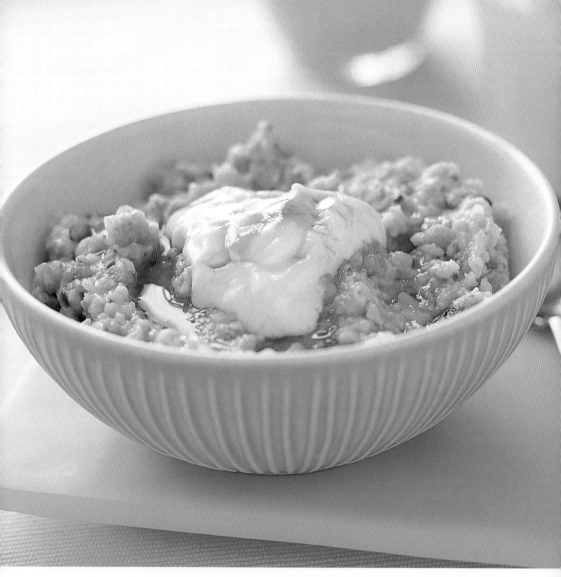

PORRIDGE IS A SUSTAINING
BREAKFAST AND ESPECIALLY NICE
ON A COLD WINTER'S MORNING.
THIS IS MADE WITH OATS PLUS A
MIXTURE OF OTHER NUTRITIOUS
GRAINS AND SEEDS, WHICH ADD
EXTRA FLAVOUR AND FIBRE.

nutrition per serve: Energy 979 kJ (234 Cal)
Fat 4.2 g
Saturated fat 0.7 g
Protein 6.4 g
Carbohydrate 40.4 g
Fibre 5.4 g
Cholesterol 0 mg

ORCHARD FRUIT COMPOTE

THIS AROMATIC FRUIT COMPOTE IS LOW GI AND A GREAT SOURCE OF FIBRE, AND WILL HELP KEEP YOU FULL AND ALERT THROUGHOUT THE MORNING. THE COMPOTE CAN ALSO BE SERVED FOR DESSERT OR AS A SNACK.

90 g (3¼ oz/¼ cup) honey

½ tsp ground ginger

1 cinnamon stick

3 whole cloves

pinch of ground nutmeg

750 ml (26 fl oz/3 cups) unsweetened apple juice

1 lemon

6 pitted prunes

3 dried peaches, halved

5 dates, halved and stones removed

10 dried apricots

1 lapsang souchong tea bag

2 golden delicious apples

2 beurre bosc pears

400 g (14 oz/1⅔ cups) low-fat vanilla yoghurt

PREP TIME: 15 MINUTES + 30 MINUTES REFRIGERATION

COOKING TIME: 45 MINUTES

SERVES 4

Put the honey, ginger, cinnamon stick, cloves, nutmeg and apple juice in a saucepan. Slice off a large piece of peel from the lemon and place in the pan. Squeeze the lemon to give 3 tablespoons juice, and add to the pan. Bring to the boil, stirring, then reduce the heat and simmer for 20 minutes.

Meanwhile, put the prunes, peaches, dates and apricots in a large heatproof bowl. Cover with boiling water, add the tea bag and leave to soak.

Peel and core the apples and pears, and cut into neat pieces about the same size as the dried fruits. Add to the syrup in the pan and simmer for 8–10 minutes, or until tender. Drain the dried fruit and discard the tea bag, then add the dried fruit to the pan and cook for a further 5 minutes.

Remove all the fruit from the pan with a slotted spoon, discard the lemon peel and place the fruit in a serving dish. Return the pan to the heat, bring to the boil, then reduce the heat and simmer for 6 minutes, or until the syrup has reduced by half. Pour the syrup over the fruit compote and refrigerate for 30 minutes. Serve with the yoghurt.

nutrition per serve: Energy 1825 kJ (436 Cal); Fat 0.6 g; Saturated fat 0.1; Protein 8.7 g; Carbohydrate 96.3 g; Fibre 7.9 g; Cholesterol 6 mg

FRESH FRUIT SALAD WITH GINGER LIME SYRUP

A BREAKFAST OF FRESH, TROPICAL FRUIT IS GREAT FOR THOSE WHO PREFER TO EAT A LIGHTER MEAL IN THE MORNING, AND IS A GREAT WAY TO BOOST YOUR INTAKE OF VITAMIN C AND OTHER ANTIOXIDANTS.

½ small ripe pineapple, cut into 3 cm (1¼ in) cubes
250 g (9 oz/1⅔ cups) strawberries, halved
500 g (1 lb 2 oz) peeled watermelon, cut into 3 cm (1¼ in) cubes
300 g (10½ oz) peeled rockmelon or any orange-fleshed melon, cut into 3 cm (1¼ in) cubes
½ papaya, cut into 3 cm (1¼ in) cubes

3 tbsp small mint leaves
45 g (1½ oz/¼ cup) soft brown sugar
125 ml (4 fl oz/½ cup) lime juice
2 cm (¾ in) piece fresh ginger, shredded
low-fat yoghurt, to serve

PREP TIME: 15 MINUTES
COOKING TIME: 15 MINUTES
SERVES 4

Put the fresh fruit and mint in a large bowl and gently mix together.

Put the sugar, lime juice and 125 ml (4 fl oz/½ cup) water in a small saucepan. Stir over low heat until the sugar has dissolved. Add the ginger and bring to the boil, then reduce the heat and simmer for 10 minutes, or until the syrup has reduced a little.

Leave the syrup to cool slightly, then pour over the fruit salad and refrigerate until cold. Serve topped with some yoghurt.

nutrition per serve: Energy 627 kJ (150 Cal); Fat 0.6 g; Saturated fat 0 g; Protein 2.9 g; Carbohydrate 30.1 g; Fibre 5.2 g; Cholesterol 0 mg

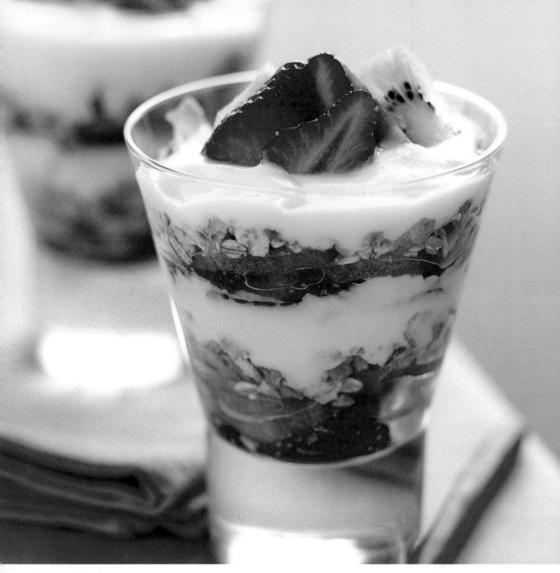

IT IS IMPORTANT TO INCLUDE
CEREALS IN OUR DAILY DIET.
THIS COLOURFUL COMBINATION
OF FRUIT, MUESLI AND YOGHURT
MAKES A REFRESHING CHANGE
FROM SERVING MUESLI WITH
PLAIN MILK.

nutrition per serve: Energy 1238 kJ (296 Cal)

Fat 4 g

Saturated fat 1 g

Protein 11.8 g

Carbohydrate 48.8 g

Fibre 7.3 g

Cholesterol 5 mg

BREAKFAST DELUXE YOGHURT

12 strawberries
4 kiwi fruit
160 g (5½ oz/1½ cups) low-fat natural
  muesli
400 g (14 oz/1⅔ cups) low-fat plain
  yoghurt
2 tbsp honey

PREP TIME: 15 MINUTES
COOKING TIME: NIL
SERVES 4

Thinly slice the strawberries. Peel and thinly slice the kiwi fruit.

Place a few slices of strawberry in the bottom of each of four glasses. Top with a few slices of kiwi fruit, then top with some muesli and yoghurt. Repeat these layers again, reserving some of the fruit, and finishing with the yoghurt. Garnish with the reserved fruit and drizzle with the honey.

HINTS:
• Use low-fat vanilla yoghurt instead of plain yoghurt, if preferred, and omit the honey.
• For a little extra fibre, top with pepitas (pumpkin seeds), dried cranberries or some ground linseeds (flax seeds).

DRIED FRUIT AND NUT QUINOA

QUINOA (PRONOUNCED AS 'KEENWA') IS A TINY LOW-GI GRAIN WITH A MILD NUTTY FLAVOUR AND SLIGHTLY CHEWY TEXTURE. IT CAN BE USED IN SWEET OR SAVOURY DISHES.

200 g (7 oz/1 cup) quinoa

500 ml (17 fl oz/2 cups) unsweetened apple juice

1 strip of orange peel

4 dried figs, chopped

4 dried peaches or dried pears, chopped

40 g (1½ oz/¼ cup) chopped raw almonds or hazelnuts

30 g (1 oz/¼ cup) pepitas (pumpkin seeds)

2 tsp grated orange zest

200 g (7 oz/1⅓ cups) strawberries, hulled and chopped

low-fat plain yoghurt, to serve

PREP TIME: 15 MINUTES
COOKING TIME: 15 MINUTES
SERVES 4–6

Put the quinoa in a sieve and rinse well under cold running water, then drain. Put the quinoa, apple juice and strip of orange peel in a saucepan.

Bring to the boil, then reduce the heat, cover and simmer for 10–15 minutes, or until all the liquid has been absorbed and the quinoa is translucent and the spiral germ ring is visible. Remove the orange peel. Cover the pan and set aside to allow the quinoa to firm up and cool a little.

Combine the dried fruit, nuts and pepitas. Add the orange zest and half the dried fruit mixture to the quinoa and stir well to combine. Spoon the mixture into four bowls and sprinkle with the remaining fruit mixture. Serve topped with the strawberries and yoghurt. Serve immediately.

HINTS:
• Quinoa can be used as a gluten-free substitute for couscous and can be found in health food shops and in the health food section of supermarkets.
• If you want to use all of the orange and not just the peel, serve with chopped orange segments instead of the strawberries.
• Use any dried fruit and nut combination in the quinoa, such as raisins, apricots, prunes and macadamias.

nutrition per serve (6): Energy 1278 kJ (305 Cal); Fat 8.1 g; Saturated fat 0.8 g; Protein 8.9 g; Carbohydrate 45.6 g; Fibre 7.1 g; Cholesterol 0 mg

SAVOURY FRENCH TOAST

THIS FRENCH TOAST IS LOWER IN FAT THAN THE REGULAR VERSION AND MAKES A SPECIAL TREAT FOR A LAZY WEEKEND. SERVE WITH SOME SPINACH AND MUSHROOMS FOR EXTRA FIBRE AND VITAMINS, IF DESIRED.

olive oil spray
4 vine-ripened tomatoes, halved
125 g (4½ oz/1 cup) grated low-fat cheddar cheese
1 small handful basil, plus extra, to garnish
8 slices soy and linseed bread

2 eggs
3 tbsp low-fat milk
25 g (1 oz) reduced-fat margarine

PREP TIME: 15 MINUTES
COOKING TIME: 20 MINUTES
SERVES 4

Spray a non-stick frying pan with oil and heat over high heat. Add the tomatoes, cut side down, and fry for 1–2 minutes until tinged with brown. Remove and keep warm in a low oven. Wipe the pan clean.

Divide the cheese and basil among four slices of the bread, then top with the remaining bread slices. Press down well to form a tight sandwich.

Beat the eggs and milk together in a wide bowl and season well with salt and pepper. Add a quarter of the margarine to the pan and heat over medium heat.

Dip the sandwiches in the egg mixture until the bread is saturated but not soggy. Drain off the excess egg mixture and cook the sandwiches for 2 minutes on each side, or until crisp and golden. (You may be able to cook two sandwiches at once, depending on the size of your pan.) Repeat with the remaining margarine and sandwiches. Cut the sandwiches in half and serve with the tomatoes.

HINT:
• Day-old bread is preferable when making French toast, as it will not absorb as much liquid as fresh bread.

nutrition per serve: Energy 1477 kJ (353 Cal); Fat 13.6 g; Saturated fat 3.6 g; Protein 28.7 g; Carbohydrate 28.2 g; Fibre 6.5 g; Cholesterol 105 mg

GRILLED STONE FRUITS WITH CINNAMON TOAST

1 tbsp reduced-fat margarine
½ tsp ground cinnamon
4 thick slices good-quality brioche
4 ripe plums, halved and stones removed
4 ripe nectarines, halved and stones
   removed

200 g (7 oz) low-fat vanilla fromage frais
2 tbsp warmed blossom honey

PREP TIME: 10 MINUTES
COOKING TIME: 10 MINUTES
SERVES 4

Put the margarine and half the cinnamon in a bowl and mix until well combined. Place the slices of brioche under a preheated grill (broiler) and grill (broil) on one side until golden. Spread the untoasted side of the brioche slices using half the cinnamon margarine, then grill until golden. Keep the toast warm in the oven.

Brush the cut side of the plums and nectarines with the remaining margarine and cook under the grill, cut side up, or in a chargrill pan, cut side down, until the fruit is tinged brown at the edges.

To serve, place two plum halves and two nectarine halves on each toasted slice of brioche. Dollop a little fromage frais on top, dust with the remaining cinnamon and drizzle with the warmed honey.

HINTS:
• Tinned plums or apricots may be used in place of the fresh stone fruits.
• For a variation on this recipe and for more fibre, serve the grilled stone fruits with toasted wholegrain fruit bread. Look for gourmet varieties of fruit bread in good delicatessens and health food shops.

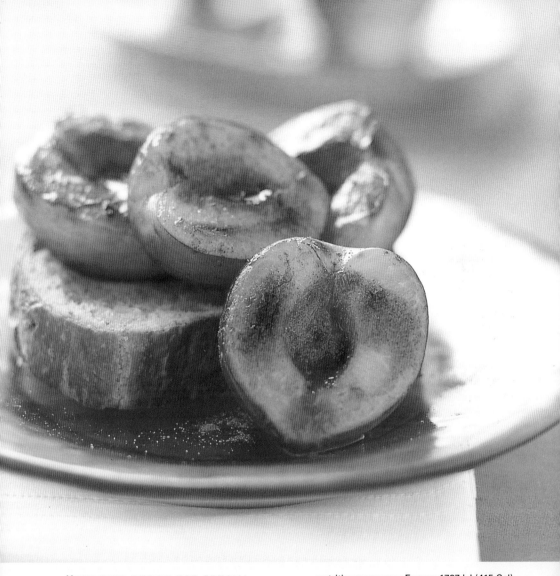

KEEP THIS RECIPE FOR SPECIAL OCCASIONS, SUCH AS A BRUNCH WITH FRIENDS, AS THE FAT IS A LITTLE TOO HIGH FOR AN EVERYDAY BREAKFAST. LEAVE THE STONE FRUIT UNPEELED FOR MAXIMUM FIBRE.

nutrition per serve: Energy 1737 kJ (415 Cal)
Fat 10.2 g
Saturated fat 4.5 g
Protein 11.7 g
Carbohydrate 65.2 g
Fibre 6.6 g
Cholesterol 42 mg

WHOLEGRAIN BAGELS WITH SPINACH AND BAKED BEANS

THIS NOURISHING BREAKFAST HAS A WONDERFUL MIX OF FLAVOURS, AND PROVIDES COMPLETE PROTEIN AND GOOD AMOUNTS OF FIBRE, AS WELL AS FOLATE, NIACIN AND BETA-CAROTENE.

425 g (15 oz) tin baked beans
200 g (7 oz/4 cups) baby English spinach
  leaves
4 wholegrain or pumpernickel bagels,
  halved
250 g (9 oz/1 cup) low-fat cottage cheese
2 tomatoes, sliced, to serve

PREP TIME: 10 MINUTES
COOKING TIME: 10 MINUTES
SERVES 4

Put the baked beans in a small saucepan and cook over medium heat for 3 minutes, or until warmed through.

Place the washed spinach in a saucepan, cover and cook over medium heat for 2 minutes, or until wilted.

Toast the bagel halves and top with the cottage cheese and spinach. Spoon the baked beans over the top and season with freshly ground black pepper. Serve with the tomato slices on the side.

HINT:
• Many large supermarkets stock different types of bagels, including wholegrain and pumpernickel varieties.

nutrition per serve: Energy 1280 kJ (306 Cal); Fat 2.3 g; Saturated fat 0.7 g; Protein 24.8 g; Carbohydrate 40.9 g; Fibre 10.3 g; Cholesterol 9 mg

SCRAMBLED EGGS WITH GRILLED TOMATOES AND MUSHROOMS

SCRAMBLED EGGS AND WHOLEGRAIN TOAST PROVIDE A NOURISHING BREAKFAST, AND THE TOMATOES, MUSHROOMS AND SPINACH ADD FLAVOUR AND NUTRIENTS.

2 vine-ripened tomatoes, halved

4 field mushrooms

canola or olive oil spray

2 tsp thyme, plus extra, to garnish

6 eggs

1 tbsp reduced-fat milk

30 g (1 oz) reduced-fat canola or olive oil margarine

4 slices wholegrain bread, toasted

50 g (1¾ oz/1 cup) baby English spinach leaves

PREP TIME: 10 MINUTES

COOKING TIME: 10 MINUTES

SERVES 2

Put the tomatoes, cut side up, and the mushrooms on a grill (broiler) tray. Spray with oil and scatter with the thyme leaves. Place the tray under a preheated grill and cook for 3–5 minutes, or until warmed.

Meanwhile, break the eggs into a bowl, add the milk and season well with salt and freshly ground black pepper. Whisk gently with a fork until well combined.

Melt half the margarine in a small non-stick saucepan or frying pan over low heat. Add the eggs, then stir constantly with a wooden spoon. Do not turn up the heat—scrambling needs to be done slowly and gently. When most of the egg has set, add the remaining margarine and remove the pan from the heat. There will be enough heat left in the pan to finish cooking the eggs and melt the margarine.

Serve the eggs immediately on toast. Arrange the tomatoes, mushrooms and spinach leaves on the side. Garnish the eggs with extra thyme.

HINT:
• It is important to use fresh eggs for scrambling. To check whether an egg is fresh, put it in a bowl of cold water. If the egg sinks on its side it is fresh; if it floats on its end it is stale. If it is somewhere between the two, the egg is not perfectly fresh but is still good enough to use.

nutrition per serve: Energy 2165 kJ (517 Cal); Fat 25.6 g; Saturated fat 6.2 g; Protein 32 g; Carbohydrate 35.3 g; Fibre 9.1 g; Cholesterol 563 mg

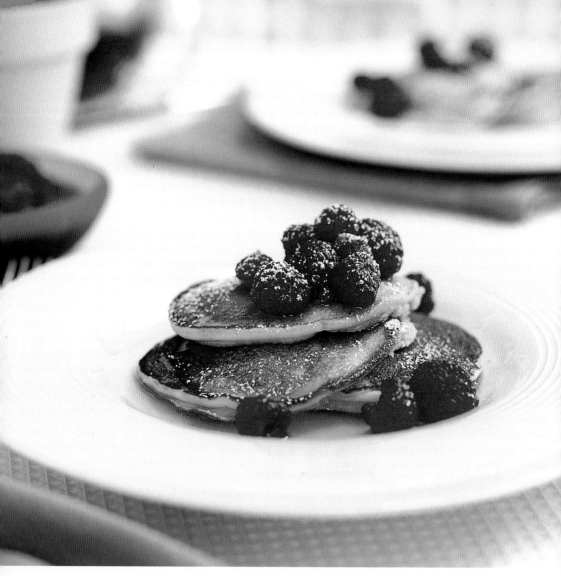

BERRIES ARE THE ULTIMATE
TREAT—THEY'RE SWEET BUT
LOW IN KILOJOULES AND
PROVIDE GOOD AMOUNTS OF
FIBRE AND ANTIOXIDANTS.

nutrition per serve (6): Energy 1286 kJ (307 Cal)
Fat 3.7 g
Saturated fat 0.5 g
Protein 11.4 g
Carbohydrate 52.8 g
Fibre 8 g
Cholesterol 0 mg

SOY PANCAKES WITH MAPLE RASPBERRIES

60 g (2¼ oz/½ cup) plain (all-purpose) flour
75 g (2½ oz/½ cup) wholemeal
  (whole-wheat) flour
50 g (1¾ oz/½ cup) soy flour
1 tbsp baking powder
2 tbsp sugar
65 g (2¼ oz) silken tofu
420 ml (14½ fl oz/1⅔ cups) low-fat soy
  milk
1 tsp natural vanilla extract

20 g (¾ oz) reduced-fat soy spread or
  margarine, melted
500 g (1 lb 2 oz/4 cups) raspberries
125 ml (4 fl oz/½ cup) pure maple syrup
icing (confectioners') sugar, for dusting

PREP TIME: 10 MINUTES + 15 MINUTES
  STANDING
COOKING TIME: 20 MINUTES
SERVES 4–6

Sift the flours, baking powder and ½ teaspoon salt into a large bowl (return the husks to the bowl), then stir in the sugar. Place the tofu, soy milk and vanilla in a food processor and combine until the mixture is smooth. Add to the dry ingredients and mix together well. Cover with plastic wrap and leave for 15 minutes.

Brush a frying pan with some of the melted spread and heat over medium heat. Cooking two pancakes at a time, drop 2 tablespoons of batter per pancake into the pan, spreading the mixture out a little with the back of the spoon. Cook for 1–2 minutes, or until bubbles form on the surface. Flip the pancake over and cook the other side for 1 minute, or until golden. Keep warm and repeat with the remaining batter to make 12 pancakes in total.

Put the raspberries and maple syrup in a saucepan and stir to combine. Gently cook for 1–2 minutes, or until the berries are warm and well coated in the syrup. Place two or three pancakes on each plate, top with the maple raspberries and dust with icing sugar.

HINTS:
• Any berries such as blackberries, blueberries or strawberries can be used instead of raspberries, if desired.
• Raspberries should be stored covered, but unwashed, in the refrigerator. Use them soon after buying them.

OMELETTE WITH ASPARAGUS, SPINACH AND SMOKED SALMON

STARTING EACH DAY WITH A HEALTHY BREAKFAST IS AN IMPORTANT HABIT FOR GOOD HEALTH. SERVE WITH A FRESHLY SQUEEZED ORANGE JUICE OR A VEGETABLE JUICE.

175 g (6 oz/1 bunch) asparagus, ends
   trimmed, cut into 5 cm (2 in) lengths
3 egg whites
3 whole eggs
1 tbsp low-fat ricotta cheese
1 tbsp chopped dill
olive oil spray
50 g (1¾ oz/1 cup) baby English spinach
   leaves

50 g (1¾ oz) smoked salmon, thinly sliced
lemon wedges, to garnish
2 slices wholegrain bread, toasted

PREP TIME: 10 MINUTES
COOKING TIME: 10 MINUTES
SERVES 2

Bring a saucepan of water to the boil. Add the asparagus and cook for 30 seconds, then remove and refresh in cold water and drain.

Whisk the egg whites in a bowl until foaming. In a separate bowl, whisk together the whole eggs and ricotta cheese, then whisk in the egg whites until well combined. Stir in the dill and season with freshly ground black pepper.

Spray a 24 cm (9½ in) non-stick frying pan with oil and heat over low heat. Pour in half the egg mixture and arrange half the asparagus pieces evenly over the top. Scatter half the spinach over the top. Cook over medium heat until the egg is just set and the spinach has started to wilt slightly. Carefully flip one half of the omelette onto the other, then transfer to a serving plate and keep warm. Repeat with the remaining egg, asparagus and spinach to make a second omelette.

Top the omelettes with smoked salmon and garnish with wedges of lemon. Serve with wholegrain toast.

nutrition per serve: Energy 1298 kJ (310 Cal); Fat 11.8 g; Saturated fat 3 g; Protein 28.3 g; Carbohydrate 20.6 g; Fibre 4 g; Cholesterol 293 mg

MIXED FRUIT FRAPPE

THIS IS AN EXCELLENT BREAKFAST DRINK, PARTICULARLY FOR THOSE WHO DON'T DRINK MILK. IT'S ALSO RICH IN HEALTHY ANTIOXIDANTS.

10 dried apricot halves
200 g (7 oz) fresh or frozen raspberries
1 banana, roughly chopped
1 mango, roughly chopped
500 ml (17 fl oz/2 cups) orange juice
1 tbsp mint leaves
6 ice cubes

PREP TIME: 5 MINUTES + 10 MINUTES
  SOAKING
COOKING TIME: NIL
SERVES 4

Put the dried apricots in a heatproof bowl. Cover with 3 tablespoons boiling water and leave to soak for 10 minutes, or until plump. Drain and roughly chop.

Blend the chopped apricots, raspberries, banana, mango, orange juice, mint and ice in a blender until thick and smooth. Do not overblend the mixture—you want to leave some small chunks of fruit. Serve immediately.

nutrition per serve: Energy 583 kJ (139 cal); Fat 0.5 g; Saturated fat 0 g; Protein 2.6 g; Carbohydrate 28.1 g; Fibre 5.2 g; Cholesterol 0 mg

VEGETABLE JUICE

1 beetroot (beet), scrubbed
10–12 carrots
2 green apples, stalks removed
2 large English spinach leaves
2 celery stalks

PREP TIME: 10 MINUTES
COOKING TIME: NIL
SERVES 2

Wash the vegetables and cut them into pieces so they will fit into your juice extractor. Juice the beetroot, carrots, apples, spinach and celery in the juice extractor.

Return some of the pulp left in the extractor to the juice (the pulp contains lots of fibre). Stir well to combine and serve chilled.

HINTS:
- When you're eating a high-fibre diet, you need to drink more fluid to help the fibre work its magic in your body, so aim to drink about 2 litres (70 fl oz/8 glasses) of fluid each day. This includes water and fluid in any other drinks and food you consume.
- The fibre content for this juice is an approximation. The more of the fibrous pulp you return to the drink, the higher the fibre content.

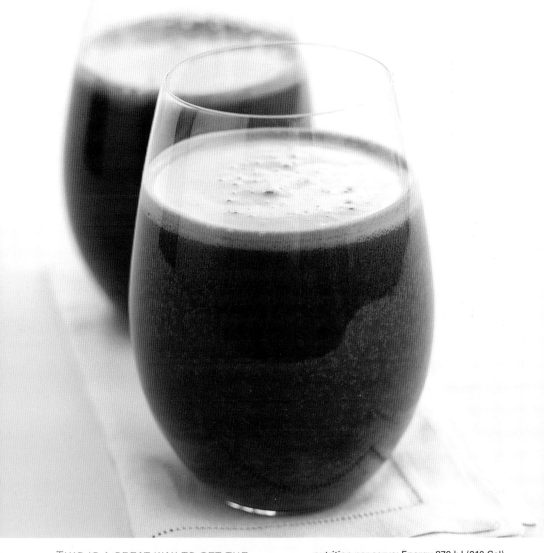

THIS IS A GREAT WAY TO GET THE
GOODNESS OF DIFFERENT-COLOURED
VEGETABLES IF YOU DON'T EAT A
VARIETY OF THEM ON A REGULAR BASIS.
THIS DRINK PACKS A NUTRITIOUS
PUNCH WITH FOLATE, POTASSIUM,
VITAMIN C AND BETA-CAROTENE.

nutrition per serve: Energy 879 kJ (210 Cal)
Fat 0.6 g
Saturated fat 0 g
Protein 4.4 g
Carbohydrate 40.1 g
Fibre 10 g
Cholesterol 0 mg

WHEAT GERM, PEACH AND BANANA SMOOTHIE

WHEAT GERM IS A HIGHLY NUTRITIOUS GRAIN, AND IS A GOOD SOURCE OF FIBRE AND FOLATE, AS WELL AS OTHER VITAMINS AND MINERALS.

375 ml (13 fl oz/1½ cups) skim milk
150 g (5½ oz/⅔ cup) low-fat vanilla
  yoghurt
2 very ripe bananas, chopped
1 large yellow peach, chopped
2 tbsp wheat germ
1 tbsp pure maple syrup

PREP TIME: 5 MINUTES
COOKING TIME: NIL
SERVES 2

Blend the milk, yoghurt, bananas, peach, wheat germ and maple syrup in a blender until combined. Do not overblend the mixture—you want to leave some small chunks of fruit. Serve immediately.

HINTS:
• If you have diabetes, omit the maple syrup, or just add a very small amount.
• You can use low-fat soy milk in this recipe. If you use soy milk, choose one that has added calcium.
• Like most other grains, wheat germ should be eaten fresh. Store in an airtight container and check the expiry date on the packet. To prolong its shelf life, you can freeze it in small portions.

nutrition per serve: Energy 1290 kJ (308 Cal); Fat 1 g; Saturated fat 0.3 g; Protein 15.5 g; Carbohydrate 57 g; Fibre 4.6 g; Cholesterol 10 mg

PLUM AND PRUNE TANG

START THE DAY THE ROUGHAGE WAY WITH THIS TANGY LOW-GI COMBO OF PLUMS AND PRUNES. USE A YOGHURT THAT CONTAINS ACIDOPHILUS CULTURE, WHICH HELPS TO MAINTAIN A HEALTHY DIGESTIVE SYSTEM.

200 g (7 oz) stoned plums, chopped
165 g (5¾ oz/¾ cup) pitted prunes,
  chopped
1 tbsp unprocessed oat bran
250 g (9 oz/1 cup) low-fat vanilla yoghurt
125 ml (4 fl oz/½ cup) buttermilk
310 ml (10¾ fl oz/1¼ cups) calcium-
  enriched skim milk
8 large ice cubes

PREP TIME: 10 MINUTES
COOKING TIME: NIL
SERVES 4

Blend the plums, prunes, oat bran, yoghurt, buttermilk, milk and ice in a blender. Don't overblend the mixture—you want to leave some small chunks of fruit. Serve immediately.

HINT:
• You can use low-fat soy milk in this recipe. If you use soy milk, choose one that has added calcium.

nutrition per serve: Energy 871 kJ (208 Cal); Fat 2.2 g; Saturated fat 1.1 g; Protein 8.8 g; Carbohydrate 35 g; Fibre 4.7 g; Cholesterol 11 mg

SALADS AND LIGHT MEALS

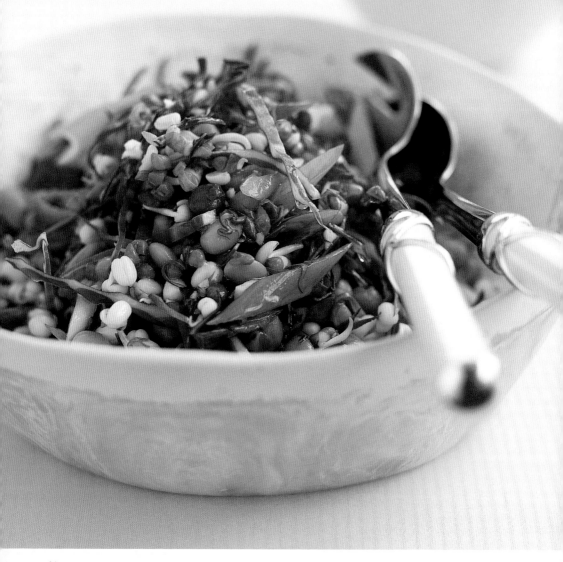

NOT ONLY A GOOD SOURCE OF FIBRE, THIS COLOURFUL AND NUTRITIOUS LOW-GI SALAD IS ALSO A GOOD SOURCE OF FOLATE AND BETA-CAROTENE. SERVE AT BARBECUES OR AS PART OF A PACKED LUNCH.

nutrition per serve: Energy 424 kJ (101 Cal)
Fat 3.4 g
Saturated fat 0.5 g
Protein 5.3 g
Carbohydrate 9.4 g
Fibre 6.2 g
Cholesterol 0 mg

54

SPROUT AND CABBAGE SALAD

½ small red cabbage (600 g/1 lb 5 oz),
   core removed, finely shredded
420 g (15 oz) tin four bean mix, drained
   and rinsed
200 g (7 oz/2¼ cups) mung bean sprouts
4 large spring onions (scallions), sliced

DRESSING
1 tbsp olive oil
2 tsp lemon juice
1 large garlic clove, crushed

PREP TIME: 15 MINUTES
COOKING TIME: NIL
SERVES 6

Put the shredded cabbage, four bean mix, bean sprouts and spring onions in a large serving bowl. Mix together gently.

To make the dressing, whisk the olive oil and lemon juice together in a small bowl. Stir in the garlic and season with salt and freshly ground black pepper. Pour the dressing over the salad and toss to combine.

HINTS:
• For extra fibre, add some sunflower seeds, pepitas (pumpkin seeds) or raw pistachio nuts to the salad.
• As a variation, wrap the salad in some pitta bread with some shredded poached chicken.
• The cabbage can be chopped, covered with plastic wrap and refrigerated for up to 3 hours before serving.

55

THREE BEAN SALAD

THIS IS A GREAT SALAD TO SERVE FOR A LARGE CROWD AT BARBECUES AND IT IS READY IN A FLASH. TINNED LEGUMES ARE A GREAT TIME-SAVER AND HAVE THE ADDED BENEFIT OF BEING HIGHLY NUTRITIOUS AND LOW GI.

250 g (9 oz) green beans, trimmed
400 g (14 oz) tin chickpeas, drained and rinsed
400 g (14 oz) tin red kidney beans, drained and rinsed
400 g (14 oz) tin cannellini beans, drained and rinsed
310 g (11 oz) tin corn kernels, drained and rinsed
3 spring onions (scallions), sliced
1 red capsicum (pepper), chopped
3 celery stalks, chopped
4–6 gherkins (pickles), chopped

3 tbsp chopped mint
3 tbsp chopped flat-leaf (Italian) parsley

MUSTARD VINAIGRETTE
125 ml (4 fl oz/½ cup) fat-free French dressing
1 tbsp dijon mustard
1 garlic clove, crushed

PREP TIME: 15 MINUTES
COOKING TIME: 2 MINUTES
SERVES 8–10

Cut the green beans into short lengths. Bring a small saucepan of water to the boil, add the beans and cook for 2 minutes. Drain and rinse under cold water, then leave in iced water until cold. Drain.

Put the green beans, chickpeas, kidney beans, cannellini beans, corn, spring onions, capsicum, celery, gherkin, mint and parsley in a large bowl. Season with salt and freshly ground black pepper and mix together.

To make the vinaigrette, put the dressing, mustard and garlic in a small bowl and whisk until well blended. Drizzle the vinaigrette over the salad and toss gently.

HINTS:
• The salad can be prepared up to 3 hours in advance and refrigerated, but don't add the dressing until just before serving.
• You can make this dish using dried beans and peas. Soak the dried beans in cold water overnight, then drain and cook in boiling water until tender. Check the packet for cooking times, as some beans take longer than others and may need to be cooked separately.

nutrition per serve (10): Energy 554 kJ (132 Cal); Fat 1.1 g; Saturated fat 0.1 g; Protein 6.8 g; Carbohydrate 20.4 g; Fibre 6.7 g; Cholesterol 0 mg

WATERCRESS, POTATO AND SALMON SALAD

THERE'S LOTS OF GOODNESS IN THIS DISH—AND IT'S DELICIOUS TOO. THERE ARE ANTIOXIDANTS, FIBRE AND EASILY ABSORBED IRON AND ZINC. SERVE WITH WHOLEGRAIN BREAD TO ADD MORE FIBRE AND CARBOHYDRATE.

150 g (5½ oz) sugar snap peas
500 g (1 lb 2 oz) kipfler (fingerling) potatoes, scrubbed
300 g (10½ oz) watercress, washed and sprigs removed
2 Lebanese (short) cucumbers, halved lengthways, sliced on the diagonal
400 g (14 oz) smoked salmon, cut into 4 cm (1½ in) pieces
3 tbsp horseradish cream

2 garlic cloves, crushed
4 tbsp light sour cream
1 tsp grated lemon zest
3 tsp lemon juice
2 tsp chopped dill

PREP TIME: 15 MINUTES
COOKING TIME: 10 MINUTES
SERVES 4

Bring a large saucepan of water to the boil. Add the snap peas and blanch them until they are bright green. Remove with a slotted spoon, refresh under cold water and set aside.

Return the water to the boil and cook the potatoes for 8–10 minutes, or until tender, then drain well. Cut into 1.5 cm (5/8 in) slices on the diagonal. Cool.

Put the sugar snap peas, potatoes, watercress, cucumbers and smoked salmon in a large bowl. Combine the horseradish, garlic, sour cream, lemon zest, lemon juice and dill in a small bowl. Spoon the dressing over the salad and toss until well combined. Season with salt and freshly ground black pepper. Serve immediately with crusty wholegrain bread.

HINT:
• To reduce the fat content, use low-fat plain yoghurt instead of sour cream.

nutrition per serve: Energy 1337 kJ (318 Cal); Fat 10 g; Saturated fat 4 g; Protein 29.8 g; Carbohydrate 23.4 g; Fibre 5.1 g; Cholesterol 59 mg

WARM CHICKEN, BEAN AND PASTA SALAD

750 g (1 lb 10 oz) orange sweet potato,
  peeled and cut into 2 cm (¾ in) cubes
250 g (9 oz) cherry tomatoes, halved
olive oil spray
2 x 200 g (7 oz) boneless, skinless chicken
  breasts
350 g (12 oz/2 bunches) asparagus,
  trimmed and cut into thirds
375 g (13 oz) macaroni

400 g (14 oz) tin cannellini beans, drained
  and rinsed
3 handfuls baby rocket (arugula) leaves
3 tbsp fat-free French dressing

PREP TIME: 15 MINUTES
COOKING TIME: 1 HOUR
SERVES 6

Preheat the oven to 200°C (400°F/Gas 6). Put the sweet potato in one end of a large non-stick roasting tin and the tomatoes in the other end, cut side down. Lightly spray with oil and bake for 45 minutes, turning halfway through cooking time. Remove the tomatoes after 30 minutes.

Meanwhile, lightly spray a chargrill pan or barbecue chargrill plate with oil and heat to high. Cook the chicken for 5 minutes on each side, or until cooked through.

Bring a large saucepan of water to the boil. Add the asparagus and cook for 1 minute, then remove with a slotted spoon and place into iced water. Drain. Return the water to the boil and cook the macaroni for 10 minutes, or until tender. Drain and keep warm.

Slice the chicken into 1 cm (½ in) thick strips and place in a large bowl with the roasted sweet potato and tomatoes, asparagus, pasta, beans and rocket and toss until combined. Add the dressing to the salad and toss until well combined. Season with salt and freshly ground black pepper and serve immediately.

HINTS:
• You can use any short pasta in this recipe, or try it with wholemeal (whole-wheat) pasta for extra fibre. Cook according to the manufacturer's directions.
• For variation, substitute the cannellini beans with tinned red kidney beans, soya beans or chickpeas.

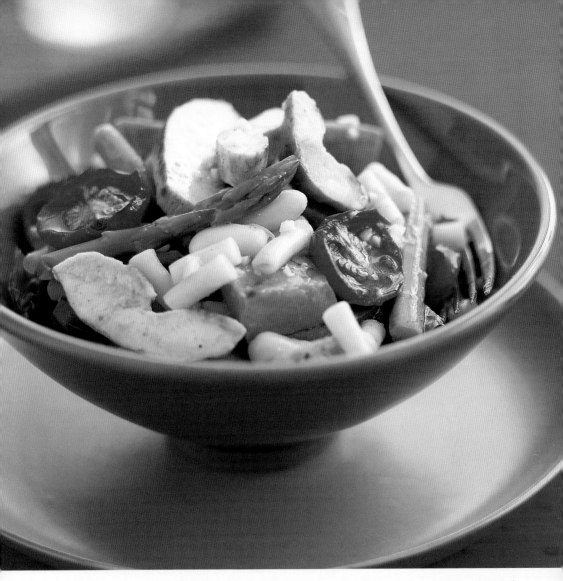

THIS IS A DELICIOUS AND NOURISHING
SALAD THAT IS LOW GI AND A GOOD
SOURCE OF FIBRE. NATURAL FIBRE-
RICH FOODS, SUCH AS PASTA,
VEGETABLES AND LEGUMES, ARE A
GREAT WAY TO MAKE LIGHT MEALS
MORE NUTRITIOUS WITHOUT ADDING
MANY KILOJOULES.

nutrition per serve: Energy 1857 kJ (444 Cal)
Fat 2.8 g
Saturated fat 0.7 g
Protein 29.3 g
Carbohydrate 70.4 g
Fibre 8.8 g
Cholesterol 47 mg

59

GRILLED TUNA AND CANNELLINI BEAN SALAD

THIS TUNA SALAD CONTAINS THE SATISFYING COMBINATION OF FISH PROTEIN, FIBRE AND LOW-GI CARBOHYDRATE FROM THE BEANS—GREAT IF YOU'RE WATCHING YOUR WEIGHT AS WELL AS YOUR FIBRE INTAKE.

400 g (14 oz) tuna steaks
cracked black pepper
1 small red onion, thinly sliced
1 tomato, seeded and chopped
1 small red capsicum (pepper), thinly sliced
2 x 400 g (14 oz) tins cannellini beans, drained and rinsed
2 garlic cloves, crushed

1 tsp chopped thyme
4 tbsp finely chopped flat-leaf (Italian) parsley
4 tbsp fat-free French dressing
100 g (3½ oz) rocket (arugula) leaves

PREP TIME: 25 MINUTES
COOKING TIME: 2 MINUTES
SERVES 4–6

Put the tuna steaks on a plate, sprinkle with cracked black pepper on both sides, cover with plastic wrap and refrigerate until needed.

Combine the onion, tomato, capsicum and cannellini beans in a large bowl. Add the garlic, thyme and 3 tablespoons of the parsley and toss to combine.

Lightly oil a barbecue chargrill plate or hotplate and heat to high. Add the tuna and cook for 1 minute on each side. The tuna should still be pink in the middle. Cut the tuna into small cubes and combine with the salad. Pour over the dressing and toss to coat.

Arrange the rocket on a platter. Top with the tuna and bean salad, season with salt and freshly ground black pepper and sprinkle with the remaining parsley.

nutrition per serve (6): Energy 848 kJ (202 Cal); Fat 4.4 g; Saturated fat 1.6 g; Protein 24.9 g; Carbohydrate 16.6 g; Fibre 7.1 g; Cholesterol 24 mg

THAI BEEF SALAD WITH MINT AND CORIANDER

PERFECT FOR A SUMMER LUNCH, THIS THAI SALAD CONTAINS A GREAT VARIETY OF COLOURFUL VEGETABLES.

2 tbsp dried shrimp

200 g (7 oz) mixed lettuce leaves

2 tsp sesame oil

500 g (1 lb 2 oz) rump steak, trimmed

90 g (3¼ oz/1 cup) bean sprouts

1 small red onion, thinly sliced

1 red capsicum (pepper), cut into thin strips

1 Lebanese (short) cucumber, cut into thin strips

200 g (7 oz) daikon radish, peeled and cut into thin strips

250 g (9 oz) cherry tomatoes, halved

1 small handful mint

1 handful coriander (cilantro) leaves

1 handful Thai basil

2 garlic cloves, finely chopped

2 tbsp chopped toasted peanuts

DRESSING

3 tbsp lime juice

3 tbsp fish sauce

1 tbsp finely chopped lemon grass

1 red chilli, seeded and chopped

1 long green chilli, seeded and chopped

1 tsp sugar

PREP TIME: 25 MINUTES + 15 MINUTES
  SOAKING

COOKING TIME: 4 MINUTES

SERVES 4

Soak the dried shrimp in hot water for 15 minutes, then drain well and finely chop. Wash the lettuce leaves and drain well.

Heat the oil in a frying pan over high heat, add the steak and cook until medium–rare, for about 1½–2 minutes on each side. Remove from the pan and leave to cool slightly. Slice the steak thinly.

To make the dressing, combine the lime juice, fish sauce, lemon grass, chillies and sugar in a small bowl. Whisk until the ingredients are combined and the sugar has dissolved.

Put the shrimp, sliced beef, bean sprouts, onion, capsicum, cucumber, radish, tomatoes, herbs and garlic in a large bowl and toss to combine. Place the salad leaves on a serving plate, top with the beef and vegetables and drizzle with the dressing, using enough of the dressing to moisten the salad. Sprinkle with the chopped peanuts.

nutrition per serve: Energy 1238 kJ (296 Cal); Fat 12.3 g; Saturated fat 3.4 g; Protein 33.8 g; Carbohydrate 9.2 g; Fibre 5.5 g; Cholesterol 81 mg

61

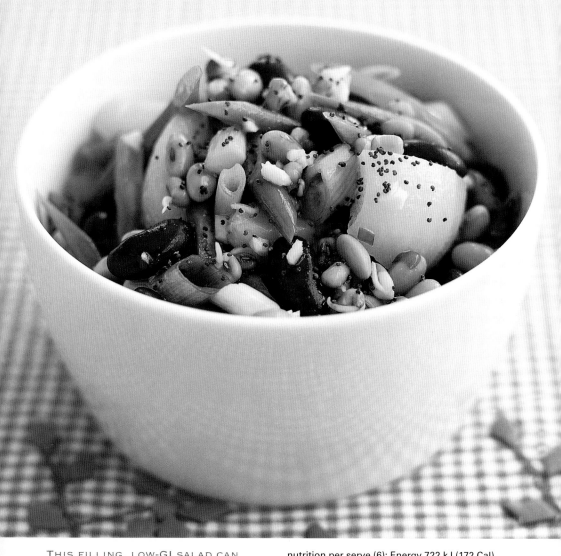

THIS FILLING, LOW-GI SALAD CAN BE SERVED AS A SIDE DISH OR AS A LIGHT MEAL. IF USING TINNED BEANS, LOOK FOR LOW-SALT VARIETIES OR TIP THE TIN INTO A SIEVE AND RINSE THE BEANS WELL TO REMOVE THE SALT.

nutrition per serve (6): Energy 722 kJ (172 Cal)

Fat 11.8 g

Saturated fat 1.6 g

Protein 4.4 g

Carbohydrate 10.6 g

Fibre 4.8 g

Cholesterol 0 mg

PEAR AND BEAN SALAD

**2 pears, unpeeled, cored and
  chopped**
45 g (1½ oz/½ cup) bean sprouts
**125 g (4½ oz/1 cup) sliced, cooked green
  beans**
4 spring onions (scallions), chopped
**125 g (4½ oz) tin red kidney beans, drained
  and rinsed**
**100 g (3½ oz/½ cup) drained and rinsed
  tinned soya beans, or use frozen**
1 tbsp poppy seeds

DRESSING
3 tbsp olive oil
1 tsp white vinegar
½ tsp sugar
1 garlic clove, crushed

PREP TIME: 20 MINUTES + 1 HOUR
   REFRIGERATION
COOKING TIME: NIL
SERVES 4–6

Combine the pears, bean sprouts, green beans, spring onions, kidney beans and soya beans in a large bowl. Mix together gently.

To make the dressing, combine the oil, vinegar, sugar, garlic and 3 tablespoons water. Taste for seasoning, then pour over the vegetables. Chill the salad for an hour before serving. Sprinkle with the poppy seeds just before you are ready to serve.

HINTS:
• You can use tinned pears instead of fresh pears if preferred, but fresh fruit with the skin left on is the better option, as most of the fibre is actually found in the skin. Just be sure to wash the fruit thoroughly before adding it to the salad.
• This salad is best made the day before serving and stored overnight in the refrigerator to enable the flavours to develop more fully.
• You can use any combination of your favourite beans.

LAMB AND BROAD BEAN PASTA SALAD

THIS PASTA SALAD IS A GOOD SOURCE OF FIBRE, FOLATE AND BETA-CAROTENE, AND THE LAMB PROVIDES SOME IRON AND ZINC. YOU CAN USE EITHER FRESH OR FROZEN BROAD BEANS.

100 g (3½ oz) sun-dried tomatoes
   (not packed in oil)
500 g (1 lb 2 oz) broad (fava) beans, to
   yield about 175 g (6 oz) podded beans
375 g (13 oz) wholemeal (whole-wheat)
   pasta
1 tablespoon olive oil
1 red onion, chopped
2 garlic cloves, lightly crushed
3 tomatoes, chopped
350 g (12 oz) lean lamb loin

100 g (3½ oz/2 cups) baby English
   spinach leaves
1 tbsp lemon juice
40 g (1½ oz/¼ cup) pine nuts,
   lightly toasted

PREP TIME: 15 MINUTES + 10 MINUTES
   SOAKING
COOKING TIME: 25 MINUTES
SERVES 6

Pour boiling water over the sun-dried tomatoes and set aside to soften for 10 minutes, then drain and chop. Peel the podded broad beans and blanch them in a saucepan of boiling water for 2 minutes. Drain and refresh in cold water.

Bring a large saucepan of water to the boil, add the pasta and cook for 12 minutes, or until *al dente*. Drain and reserve 125 ml (4 fl oz/½ cup) of pasta water.

While the pasta is cooking, heat the oil in a large frying pan, add the onion and cook for 2–3 minutes, then add the garlic and cook for a further 2 minutes. Remove to a large bowl with a slotted spoon and stir in the chopped fresh tomatoes. Reheat the pan and, when hot, add the lamb. Brown well on both sides, then cook for a further 2–3 minutes on each side until just cooked. The flesh will still be slightly pink in the centre. Cover and set aside for 5 minutes, then thinly slice the lamb on the diagonal.

Add the sun-dried tomatoes, broad beans and lamb to the onion and tomato mixture and gently combine. Toss through the hot pasta, adding the spinach, reserved water and the lemon juice. Scatter over the pine nuts and toss to combine. Divide among serving plates, season with freshly ground black pepper and serve immediately.

nutrition per serve: Energy 1848 kJ (441 Cal); Fat 12.4 g; Saturated fat 2.3 g; Protein 26.4 g; Carbohydrate 50.7 g; Fibre 12 g; Cholesterol 38 mg

FRESH BEETROOT AND GOAT'S CHEESE SALAD

FRESH BEETROOT HAS A LOVELY EARTHY SWEET FLAVOUR AND WONDERFUL COLOUR. LEAVING SOME OF THE STALK ATTACHED TO THE BULB WILL ENSURE IT DOESN'T 'BLEED' AND LOSE ITS COLOUR WHILE IT IS COOKING.

1 kg (2 lb 4 oz) beetroot (beets), with
leaves (4 bulbs)
200 g (7 oz) green beans,
trimmed
1 tbsp red wine vinegar
2 tbsp extra virgin olive oil
1 garlic clove, crushed

1 tbsp capers in brine, rinsed and roughly
chopped
100 g (3½ oz) goat's cheese

PREP TIME: 15 MINUTES
COOKING TIME: 40 MINUTES
SERVES 4

Trim the leaves from the beetroot, leaving about 3 cm (1¼ in) of stalk attached to the bulb. Scrub the bulbs and wash the leaves well. Bring a large saucepan of water to the boil, add the beetroot, then reduce the heat and simmer, covered, for 30 minutes, or until tender when pierced with a knife. (The cooking time may vary depending on the size of the bulbs.) Drain and cool. Peel the skins off the beetroot and cut the bulbs into wedges.

Meanwhile, bring a saucepan of water to the boil, add the beans and cook for 3 minutes, or until just tender. Remove with tongs and place in a bowl of cold water. Drain well. Add the beetroot leaves to the boiled water and cook for 3–5 minutes over medium heat until the leaves and stems are tender. Drain, transfer to a bowl of cold water, then drain well.

To make the dressing, put the vinegar, oil, garlic, capers and ½ teaspoon freshly ground black pepper into a screw-top jar and shake well. Taste for seasoning. To serve, divide the beans and beetroot wedges and leaves among four serving plates. Crumble the goat's cheese over the top and drizzle with the dressing.

HINTS:
• The beetroot cooking time will vary depending on the size of the bulb. Small bulbs take 30 minutes, medium will take about 45 minutes, and large bulbs may take 60 minutes.
• You can use feta cheese instead of goat's cheese, if preferred. Using reduced- or low-fat feta or goat's cheese will lower the fat content further.

nutrition per serve: Energy 954 kJ (228 Cal); Fat 13.4 g; Saturated fat 3.9 g; Protein 7.8 g; Carbohydrate 15.9 g; Fibre 7.1 g; Cholesterol 10 mg

BEAN ENCHILADAS

1 tbsp light olive oil
1 onion, thinly sliced
3 garlic cloves, crushed
1 bird's eye chilli, finely chopped
2 tsp ground cumin
125 ml (4 fl oz/½ cup) vegetable stock
3 tomatoes, peeled, seeded and chopped
   (see Hint)
1 tbsp tomato paste (concentrated purée)
2 x 420 g (15 oz) tins three bean mix,
   drained and rinsed

2 tbsp chopped coriander (cilantro) leaves
8 flour tortillas
1 small avocado, chopped
125 g (4½ oz/½ cup) light sour cream
1 handful coriander (cilantro) sprigs
115 g (4 oz/2 cups) shredded lettuce

PREP TIME: 20 MINUTES
COOKING TIME: 20 MINUTES
MAKES 8

Heat the olive oil in a deep frying pan over medium heat. Add the onion and cook for 3–4 minutes, or until just soft. Add the garlic and chilli and cook for a further 30 seconds. Add the cumin, stock, tomatoes and tomato paste and cook for 6–8 minutes, or until the mixture is quite thick and pulpy. Season with salt and freshly ground black pepper.

Preheat the oven to 170°C (325°F/Gas 3). Add the bean mix to the sauce and cook for 5 minutes to heat through, then add the chopped coriander.

Meanwhile, wrap the tortillas in foil and warm in the oven for 3–4 minutes.

Place a warm tortilla on a plate and spread with some of the bean mixture. Top with some avocado, sour cream, coriander sprigs and lettuce. Roll the enchiladas up, tucking in the ends. Cut each one in half to serve.

HINT:
• To peel the tomatoes, score a cross in the base of each tomato. Put in a heatproof bowl and cover with boiling water. Leave for 30 seconds, then transfer to cold water and peel the skin away from the cross. To seed, cut the tomato in half and scoop out the seeds with a teaspoon.

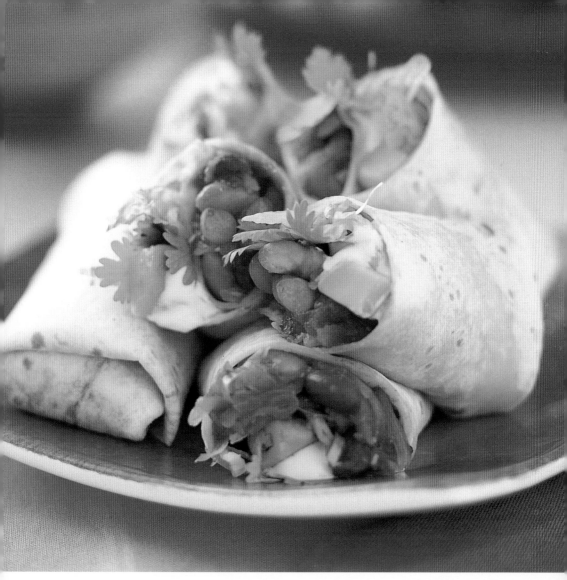

THESE BEAN ENCHILADAS ARE
QUITE FILLING, SO FOR A LIGHT
MEAL OR SNACK YOU MAY ONLY
WANT TO EAT ONE, AND SERVE
IT WITH A MIXED LEAF SALAD.
FOR A MAIN MEAL, SERVE TWO
PER PERSON.

nutrition per enchilada: Energy 993 kJ (237 Cal)
Fat 11.1 g
Saturated fat 2.8 g
Protein 8.5 g
Carbohydrate 22.8 g
Fibre 6.5 g
Cholesterol 10 mg

67

VEGETARIAN RICE PAPER ROLLS

THIS VEGETARIAN SNACK IS FULL OF VITAMIN C, BETA-CAROTENE AND FOLATE, AND MAKES GREAT FINGER FOOD FOR PARTIES. LEAVE THE VEGETABLES UNPEELED FOR EXTRA FIBRE.

50 g (1¾ oz) dried rice vermicelli
200 g (7 oz) frozen soya beans
16 square (15 cm/6 in) rice paper wrappers
1 zucchini (courgette), cut into thin
    matchsticks
1 Lebanese (short) cucumber, cut into thin
    matchsticks
1 carrot, grated
1 large handful mint, finely shredded
100 g (3½ oz) firm tofu, cut into 1 cm
    (½ in) wide batons

DIPPING SAUCE
80 ml (2½ fl oz/⅓ cup) fish sauce
2 tbsp chopped coriander (cilantro) leaves
2 small red chillies, finely chopped
2 tsp soft brown sugar
2 tsp lime juice

PREP TIME: 40 MINUTES + 5 MINUTES
    SOAKING
COOKING TIME: 2 MINUTES
SERVES 4

Soak the vermicelli in hot water for 5 minutes, or until soft. Drain and cut into 5 cm (2 in) lengths using scissors. Bring a saucepan of water to the boil, add the soya beans and cook for 2 minutes, then drain well.

Working with no more than two wrappers at a time, dip each rice paper wrapper in warm water for 10 seconds. Remove from the water and lay out on a flat work surface.

Place a small amount of vermicelli noodles on the bottom third of each wrapper, leaving a 2 cm (¾ in) border either side. Top with some zucchini, cucumber, carrot, soya beans, mint and two batons of tofu. Keeping the filling compact and neat, fold in the sides and roll up tightly. Seal with a little water. Cover with a damp cloth while you assemble the remaining rolls.

To make the dipping sauce, combine the fish sauce, coriander, chilli, sugar, lime juice and 2 tablespoons water in a small bowl. Serve with the rice paper rolls.

nutrition per serve: Energy 1284 kJ (307 Cal); Fat 5.7 g; Saturated fat 0.7 g; Protein 15.1 g; Carbohydrate 46.5 g; Fibre 5 g; Cholesterol 0 mg

DAL

WE NEED TO INCLUDE BOTH SOLUBLE AND INSOLUBLE FIBRE IN OUR DIET, AND LENTILS ARE A GREAT SOURCE OF SOLUBLE FIBRE. THIS DISH CAN BE SERVED WITH RICE AND VEGETABLES AS A COMPLETE VEGETARIAN MEAL.

200 g (7 oz/1 cup) red lentils
¼ tsp ground turmeric
1 tbsp oil
½ tsp brown mustard seeds
1 tbsp cumin seeds
1 onion, finely chopped
1 tbsp grated fresh ginger
2 long green chillies, halved lengthways

80 ml (2½ fl oz/⅓ cup) lemon juice
2 tbsp finely chopped coriander (cilantro) leaves

PREP TIME: 10 MINUTES

COOKING TIME: 40 MINUTES

SERVES 6

Put the lentils in a saucepan, cover with 750 ml (26 fl oz/3 cups) water and bring to the boil. Reduce the heat, stir in the turmeric, then cover and simmer for 20 minutes, or until the lentils are tender.

Heat the oil in a saucepan, add the mustard and cumin seeds and cook until the mustard seeds begin to pop. Add the onion, ginger and chillies and cook for 5 minutes, or until the onion is golden.

Add the lentils and 125 ml (4 fl oz/½ cup) water to the pan. Season with salt, reduce the heat and simmer for 10 minutes. Remove from the heat, stir in the lemon juice and garnish with the coriander. Serve with naan breads, or as part of a vegetarian meal with rice and curried vegetables.

nutrition per serve: Energy 585 kJ (140 Cal); Fat 4 g; Saturated fat 0.5 g; Protein 8.8 g; Carbohydrate 14.9 g; Fibre 5.3 g; Cholesterol 0 mg

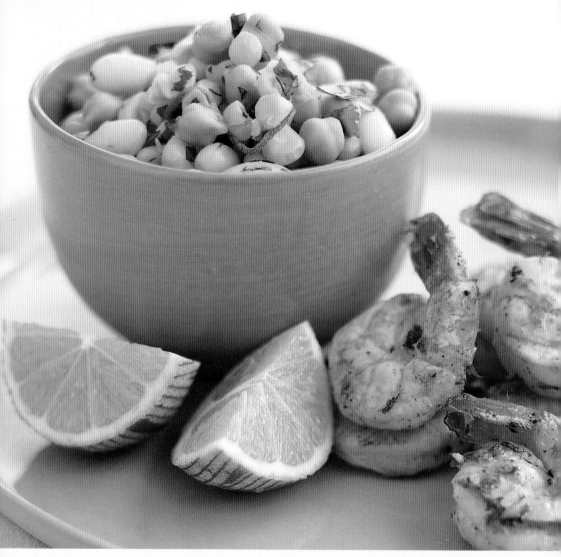

PRAWNS PROVIDE MINERALS AND
PROTEIN WITH RELATIVELY FEW
KILOJOULES—A GREAT CHOICE FOR
THOSE WATCHING THEIR WEIGHT.
THE LOW-GI SALSA IS A GOOD
SOURCE OF FIBRE AND FOLATE.

nutrition per serve: Energy 1139 kJ (272 Cal)
Fat 7.3 g
Saturated fat 1.1 g
Protein 23.4 g
Carbohydrate 24.6 g
Fibre 8.3 g
Cholesterol 101 mg

MARINATED PRAWNS WITH CORN AND CHICKPEA SALSA

400 g (14 oz) tin cannellini beans, drained
and rinsed
300 g (10½ oz) tin chickpeas, drained
and rinsed
310 g (11 oz) tin corn kernels, drained
and rinsed
1 tsp grated lime zest
2 tbsp chopped coriander (cilantro) leaves
500 g (1 lb 2 oz) large raw prawns (shrimp)
2 tbsp lemon juice

1 tbsp sesame oil
2 garlic cloves, crushed
2 tsp grated fresh ginger
canola or olive oil spray
lime wedges, to serve

PREP TIME: 15 MINUTES + 3 HOURS
MARINATING
COOKING TIME: 5 MINUTES
SERVES 4

Combine the cannellini beans, chickpeas and corn kernels in a large bowl. Stir in the lime zest and coriander.

Peel the prawns, leaving the tails intact. Gently pull out the dark vein from each prawn back, starting at the head end.

To make the marinade, combine the lemon juice, sesame oil, garlic and ginger in a small bowl. Add the prawns and gently stir to coat them in the marinade. Cover and refrigerate for at least 3 hours.

Lightly spray a barbecue hotplate with oil and heat to high. Add the prawns and cook for 3–5 minutes, or until pink and cooked through. Brush frequently with the marinade while cooking. Serve immediately with the corn, bean and chickpea salsa and wedges of lime.

HINTS:
• Alternatively, the prawns can be threaded onto bamboo skewers. To prepare the skewers, soak them in cold water for about 30 minutes, which will prevent the skewers burning during cooking. After marinating, thread the prawns evenly onto the skewers and cook as stated, turning and basting occasionally during cooking.
• The salsa can be served as a side dish to any barbecued seafood or meat.

PIZZETTE

MAKING YOUR OWN PIZZAS MEANS YOU CAN ENJOY THEM WITH LESS FAT THAN COMMERCIAL VARIETIES. BY USING WHOLEMEAL FLOUR INSTEAD OF WHITE FOR THE CRUST, YOU GET MORE FIBRE AND B-GROUP VITAMINS.

300 g (10½ oz/2 cups) wholemeal
　(whole-wheat) flour
2 tsp dry yeast
½ tsp sugar
2 tbsp plain yoghurt

TOPPING
2 tbsp tomato paste (concentrated purée)
1 garlic clove, crushed
1 tsp dried oregano
80 g (2¾ oz) lean shaved ham, sliced
　into strips

2 tbsp grated light mozzarella cheese
20 g (¾ oz) baby rocket (arugula) leaves,
　torn
extra virgin olive oil, to drizzle

PREP TIME: 10 MINUTES + 20–30 MINUTES
　STANDING
COOKING TIME: 12–15 MINUTES
SERVES 4

Sift the flour into a bowl, then return the husks to the bowl. Add the yeast, sugar and ½ teaspoon salt. Make a well in the centre, add 125 ml (4 fl oz/½ cup) water and the yoghurt and mix to form a dough.

Knead on a lightly floured surface for 5 minutes, or until smooth and elastic. Place the dough in a lightly oiled bowl, cover with a tea towel (dish towel) and rest in a warm place for 20–30 minutes, or until doubled in size. Preheat the oven to 200ºC (400°F/Gas 6).

Punch the dough down and knead for 30 seconds, then divide into four portions. Roll each portion into a 15 cm (6 in) round and place on a baking tray.

To make the topping, combine the tomato paste, garlic, oregano and 1 tablespoon water. Spread the paste over each base, then top each with some shaved ham and mozzarella. Bake for 12–15 minutes, or until crisp and golden on the edges. Just before serving, top with the torn rocket and drizzle with extra virgin olive oil. Serve with a vinegar-dressed mixed leaf salad, if desired.

nutrition per serve: Energy 1347 kJ (322 Cal); Fat 4.7 g; Saturated fat 1.4 g; Protein 15.8 g; Carbohydrate 49.2 g; Fibre 9.4 g; Cholesterol 15 mg

WHOLEGRAIN TUNA MAYONNAISE SANDWICHES

FOR GOOD HEALTH, IT'S IMPORTANT TO EAT THREE TO FOUR SERVES OF OMEGA-3-RICH FISH EACH WEEK. THE WHOLEGRAIN BREAD PROVIDES SOLUBLE AND INSOLUBLE FIBRE, AS WELL AS SOME RESISTANT STARCH.

210 g (7½ oz) tin tuna in spring water, drained
1 carrot, grated
2 spring onions (scallions), finely chopped
90 g (3¼ oz/⅓ cup) low-fat mayonnaise
1 coral lettuce, washed and drained
8 large slices dense wholegrain bread
4 gherkins (pickles), thinly sliced

PREP TIME: 15 MINUTES
COOKING TIME: NIL
SERVES 4

Put the tuna in a small bowl with the carrot, spring onion and mayonnaise and mix to combine. Divide the lettuce leaves among four slices of bread. Top with the tuna and mayonnaise mixture and the gherkins.

Season to taste with salt and freshly ground black pepper. Top with the remaining four slices of bread.

HINT:
• Look for good-quality wholegrain breads in supermarkets and bakeries. Wholegrain breads have a high fibre content and contain a combination of healthy grains and seeds. The more grains in the bread, the more fibre and resistant starch it contains.

nutrition per serve: Energy 1366 kJ (326 Cal); Fat 6 g; Saturated fat 1.3 g; Protein 22.8 g; Carbohydrate 38 g; Fibre 13.5 g; Cholesterol 20 mg

VEGETABLE FRITTATA

2 large red capsicums (peppers)
500 g (1 lb 2 oz) eggplant (aubergine), cut into 1 cm (½ in) slices
olive oil spray
600 g (1 lb 5 oz) orange sweet potato, peeled and cut into 1 cm (½ in) slices
2 tsp olive oil
2 leeks, white part only, thinly sliced
2 garlic cloves, crushed
250 g (9 oz) zucchini (courgette), thinly sliced

8 eggs, lightly beaten
2 tbsp finely chopped basil
70 g (2½ oz/¾ cup) grated parmesan cheese
200 g (7 oz) reduced-fat hummus
baby rocket (arugula) leaves, to serve

PREP TIME: 30 MINUTES
COOKING TIME: 40 MINUTES
SERVES 6

Cut the capsicums into large flat pieces, removing the seeds and membranes. Put the capsicums, skin side up, under a preheated grill (broiler) until the skin blackens. Leave covered under a tea towel (dish towel) until cool, then peel away the skin.

Arrange the eggplant slices in a single layer on the grill tray. Spray with oil and grill (broil) for 2–3 minutes. Turn the eggplant slices over and respray with oil, cooking for a further 2–3 minutes, or until softened. Drain on paper towels.

Cook the sweet potato in a saucepan of boiling water for 4–5 minutes, or until just tender, then drain well.

Heat the oil in a deep round 23 cm (9 in) frying pan over medium heat. Add the leek and garlic and stir for 1 minute, or until soft. Add the zucchini and cook for 2 minutes, then remove from the pan.

Line the base of the pan with half the eggplant and top with the leek mixture. Cover with the roasted capsicum, then with the remaining eggplant and finally the sweet potato.

Put the eggs, basil and parmesan in a bowl and season with freshly ground black pepper. Mix well and pour over the vegetables in the pan. Cook over low heat for 15 minutes, or until almost cooked. Place the pan under a hot grill for 2–3 minutes, or until the top of the frittata is golden and cooked. Cut into six wedges. Serve with hummus and rocket.

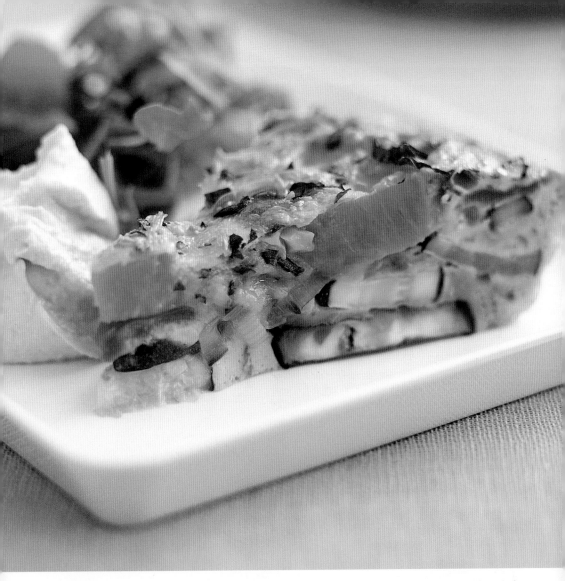

THIS COLOURFUL AND NOURISHING
FRITTATA IS GREAT FOR LUNCH OR
A LIGHT DINNER, OR CAN BE EATEN
COLD FOR PICNICS OR PACKED
LUNCHES. SERVE WITH FRESH
GRAINY BREAD OR PUMPERNICKEL
BREAD FOR A FIBRE-RICH MEAL.

nutrition per serve: Energy 1309 kJ (313 Cal)
Fat 14.8 g
Saturated fat 4.8 g
Protein 19.1 g
Carbohydrate 23.2 g
Fibre 7.4 g
Cholesterol 260 mg

BAKED SWEET POTATO AND LENTIL RISSOLES

BIG ON FLAVOUR AND LOW IN FAT, THESE MILDLY SPICY RISSOLES ARE RICH IN CARBOHYDRATE AND FIBRE AND PROVIDE GOOD AMOUNTS OF FOLATE, BETA-CAROTENE AND NIACIN.

400 g (14 oz) tin brown lentils, drained and rinsed
1 small onion, finely chopped
1 small green capsicum (pepper), finely chopped
1 carrot, grated
2 tbsp chopped flat-leaf (Italian) parsley
425 g (15 oz/1⅓ cups) cooked and mashed sweet potato
160 g (5½ oz/2 cups) fresh wholegrain breadcrumbs (2–3 slices bread)
1 tsp ground cumin
dry wholegrain breadcrumbs, for coating
olive oil spray

SAUCE
185 ml (6 fl oz/¾ cup) tomato sauce (ketchup)
1–2 tsp curry powder
2 tsp lemon juice

PREP TIME: 20 MINUTES + 30 MINUTES REFRIGERATION
COOKING TIME: 40 MINUTES
SERVES 4

Combine the lentils, onion, capsicum, carrot and parsley in a large bowl. Use clean hands to combine and then mix in the mashed sweet potato, breadcrumbs and cumin. Season well with salt and freshly ground black pepper. Divide the mixture into eight even-sized patties and refrigerate for at least 30 minutes to firm up and develop flavour.

Preheat the oven to 200°C (400°F/Gas 6). Line a baking tray with baking paper.

Coat the rissoles in the dry breadcrumbs and spray the rissoles with the oil. Place on the prepared tray and bake, turning once or twice, for 35 minutes, or until crisp and golden.

Meanwhile, combine the sauce ingredients in a small saucepan and bring just to the boil. Set aside. Serve the rissoles hot or cold with the tomato sauce and a mixed salad.

nutrition per serve: Energy 1475 kJ (352 Cal); Fat 6.8 g; Saturated fat 0.8 g; Protein 11.5 g; Carbohydrate 57.1 g; Fibre 9 g; Cholesterol 0 mg

ROAST VEGETABLE QUICHE

THIS QUICHE CONTAINS A GREAT VARIETY OF HEALTHY VEGETABLES. SERVE WITH A SALAD AND SOME WHOLEGRAIN BREAD.

1 large potato, unpeeled

400 g (14 oz) peeled pumpkin (winter squash)

200 g (7 oz) orange sweet potato, unpeeled

2 large parsnips, unpeeled

1 red capsicum (pepper)

2 onions, cut into wedges

6 garlic cloves, halved

2 tsp olive oil

90 g (3¼ oz/¾ cup) plain (all-purpose) flour

75 g (2½ oz/½ cup) wholemeal (whole-wheat) flour

40 g (1½ oz) reduced-fat margarine

45 g (1½ oz) ricotta cheese

250 ml (9 fl oz/1 cup) skim milk

3 eggs, lightly beaten

30 g (1 oz/¼ cup) grated reduced-fat cheddar cheese

2 tbsp chopped basil

PREP TIME: 45 MINUTES + 25 MINUTES
REFRIGERATION

COOKING TIME: 2½ HOURS

SERVES 6

Preheat the oven to 180°C (350°F/Gas 4). Lightly grease a 3.5 cm (1¼ in) deep, 23 cm (9 in) loose-based flan tin.

Cut the potato, pumpkin, sweet potato, parsnips and capsicum into bite-sized chunks, place in a roasting tin with the onion and garlic and drizzle with the oil. Season and bake for 1 hour, or until the vegetables are tender. Leave to cool.

Mix the flours, margarine and ricotta cheese in a food processor, then slowly add up to 3 tablespoons of the milk, or enough to form a soft dough. Turn out onto a lightly floured surface and gather together into a smooth ball. Cover and refrigerate for 15 minutes.

Roll the pastry out on a lightly floured surface, then ease into the tin, bringing it gently up the side of the tin. Trim the edge and refrigerate for 10 minutes. Increase the oven to 200°C (400°F/Gas 6). Cover the pastry with crumpled baking paper and fill with baking beads or uncooked rice. Bake for 10 minutes, remove the beads and paper, then bake for another 10 minutes, or until golden brown.

Place the vegetables in the pastry base and pour in the combined remaining milk, eggs, cheese and basil. Reduce the oven to 180°C (350°F/Gas 4) and bake for 1 hour 10 minutes, or until set in the centre. Leave for 5 minutes before removing from the tin to serve.

nutrition per serve: Energy 1313 kJ (314 Cal); Fat 9.5 g; Saturated fat 2.9 g; Protein 14.4 g; Carbohydrate 39.6 g; Fibre 5.9 g; Cholesterol 102 mg

77

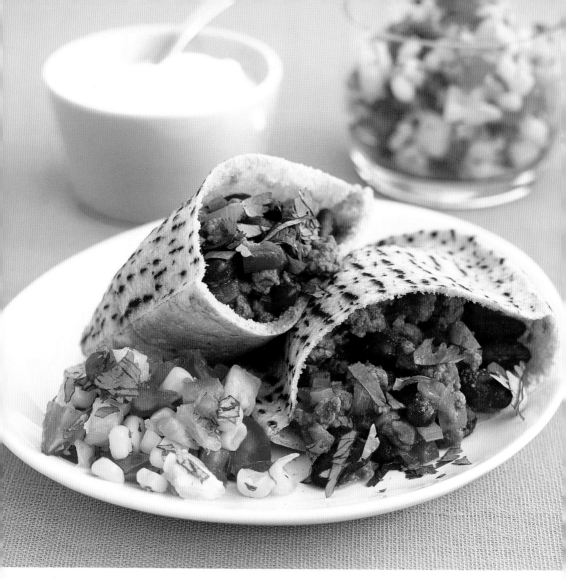

A MORE NUTRITIOUS SUBSTITUTE
FOR TAKEAWAY PIZZAS OR MEXICAN
FOOD, THIS QUICK MEAL PROVIDES
PROTEIN, IRON AND ZINC, AND IS
AN EXCELLENT SOURCE OF FIBRE.

nutrition per serve: Energy 2400 kJ (573 Cal)
Fat 11.1 g
Saturated fat 3.5 g
Protein 38.8 g
Carbohydrate 70.1 g
Fibre 14.8 g
Cholesterol 54 mg

BEEF PITTAS WITH PINEAPPLE SALSA

1 tsp olive oil
1 onion, finely chopped
1 celery stalk, finely chopped
½ red capsicum (pepper), finely chopped
400 g (14 oz) lean minced (ground) beef
1 tsp ground cumin
½ tsp ground coriander
1 tbsp tomato paste (concentrated purée)
250 g (9 oz/1 cup) bottled tomato pasta
 sauce
240 g (8½ oz) tinned red kidney beans,
 drained and rinsed
4 wholemeal (whole-wheat) pitta
 breads
250 g (9 oz/1 cup) low-fat plain yoghurt

PINEAPPLE SALSA
½ pineapple
4 vine-ripened tomatoes
310 g (11 oz) tin corn kernels, drained and
 rinsed
50 g (1¾ oz/½ large bunch) coriander
 (cilantro) leaves, chopped
1 tbsp lemon juice

PREP TIME: 15 MINUTES

COOKING TIME: 20 MINUTES

SERVES 4

Heat the oil in a large, non-stick frying pan. Add the onion, celery and capsicum and cook, stirring, for 2 minutes, or until softened. Increase the heat, add the beef and cook for 5 minutes, or until the meat changes colour. Break up any lumps with a fork. Stir in the cumin, coriander and tomato paste. Add the pasta sauce and 125 ml (4 fl oz/½ cup) water. Simmer and stir frequently for 8 minutes, or until cooked and slightly reduced. Stir in the kidney beans.

To make the pineapple salsa, peel and finely chop the pineapple. Cut the tomatoes into quarters, remove the seeds with a spoon, and finely chop the flesh. Combine the salsa ingredients, reserving half of the coriander leaves for garnish.

Preheat the oven to 180°C (350°F/Gas 4). Wrap the pitta breads in foil and warm them in the oven for 5 minutes.

To serve, cut the pitta breads in half, fill with the beef and bean mixture and top with the yoghurt. Sprinkle with the reserved coriander and serve with the salsa.

BAKED SWEET POTATOES WITH AVOCADO AND CORN SALSA

A SATISFYING SNACK OR LIGHT MEAL, THIS COLOURFUL DISH IS A NUTRITIOUS TREAT FOR CHILDREN, PROVIDING MONOUNSATURATED FAT, ANTIOXIDANTS AND FIBRE.

4 x 200 g (7 oz) orange sweet potatoes, unpeeled
1 red onion, finely chopped
1 avocado, finely chopped
1 tbsp lemon juice
125 g (4½ oz) tin corn kernels, drained and rinsed
½ red capsicum (pepper), finely chopped

1 tbsp sweet chilli sauce
2 tbsp light sour cream or low-fat plain yoghurt
2 tbsp chopped flat-leaf (Italian) parsley

PREP TIME: 15 MINUTES
COOKING TIME: 40 MINUTES
SERVES 4

Preheat the oven to 200°C (400°F/Gas 6). Scrub the sweet potatoes clean, dry them and pierce several times with a skewer. Bake directly on the oven rack for 40 minutes, or until tender when tested with a skewer.

Meanwhile, put the onion, avocado, lemon juice, corn and capsicum in a bowl and mix together well. Stir in the chilli sauce and season with salt and freshly ground black pepper.

Make a deep cut along the top of each cooked sweet potato. Divide the topping among the sweet potatoes and add a dollop of sour cream or yoghurt to each. Sprinkle with the parsley and serve with a green salad.

nutrition per serve: Energy 1338 kJ (320 Cal); Fat 15.1 g; Saturated fat 3.6 g; Protein 6.7 g; Carbohydrate 36.5 g; Fibre 5.7 g; Cholesterol 6 mg

TABOULEH AND HUMMUS POTATOES

POTATOES HAVE MANY NUTRITIONAL QUALITIES, SUCH AS BEING HIGH IN CARBOHYDRATES AND FIBRE, BUT IT'S THE TOPPINGS OF BUTTER AND SOUR CREAM THAT CAN SEND THE FAT METER SOARING. TRY THIS LOW-FAT IDEA.

4 x 200 g (7 oz) roasting potatoes,
  unpeeled
45 g (1½ oz/¼ cup) burghul (bulgar)
3 large handfuls flat-leaf (Italian) parsley,
  chopped
2 large handfuls mint, chopped
2 spring onions (scallions), thinly sliced
1 tomato, finely chopped

2 tbsp olive oil
2 tbsp lemon juice
4 tbsp reduced-fat hummus

PREP TIME: 10 MINUTES + 15 MINUTES
  SOAKING
COOKING TIME: 1 HOUR
SERVES 4

Preheat the oven to 210°C (415°F/Gas 6–7). Scrub the potatoes clean, dry them and pierce several times with a skewer. Bake directly on the oven rack for 1 hour, or until tender when tested with a skewer. Leave to stand for 2 minutes.

While the potatoes are baking, make the tabouleh. Soak the burghul in 3 tablespoons water for 15 minutes, or until all the water has been absorbed. Put in a bowl with the parsley, mint, spring onion, tomato, olive oil and lemon juice. Season well with salt and freshly ground black pepper.

Cut a large cross in the top of each cooked potato and squeeze gently from the base to open—if the potato is still too hot, hold the potato in a clean tea towel (dish towel). Spoon a tablespoon of hummus onto each potato and top with the tabouleh.

nutrition per serve: Energy 985 kJ (235 Cal); Fat 3.7 g; Saturated fat 0.5 g; Protein 8.2 g; Carbohydrate 37 g; Fibre 8.1 g; Cholesterol 0 mg

PRAWN TORTILLAS WITH MANGO SALSA

MANGO SALSA
½ red onion, finely chopped
2 mangoes, finely chopped
4 vine-ripened tomatoes, seeded and
    finely chopped
1 Lebanese (short) cucumber, peeled,
    seeded and finely chopped
1 celery stalk, thinly sliced
3 handfuls mint, chopped
2 tbsp fat-free French dressing

olive oil spray
16 raw prawns (shrimp), peeled and
    deveined, tails left intact
8 flour tortillas (20 cm/8 in)
coriander (cilantro) leaves, to serve
lemon wedges, to serve

PREP TIME: 20 MINUTES
COOKING TIME: 5 MINUTES
MAKES 8

To make the mango salsa, combine the onion, mango, tomato, cucumber, celery and mint in a large bowl. Add the dressing and toss to combine.

Lightly spray a barbecue hotplate with the oil and heat to high. Add the prawns and cook, turning occasionally, for 2–3 minutes, or until just cooked through. Wrap the tortillas in foil and place them on a warm part of the barbecue to heat through.

To serve, fold the tortillas into four. Arrange the tortillas, mango salsa and prawns on the plate and garnish with the coriander leaves. Serve with the lemon wedges.

HINTS:
• If fresh mango is not available, use tinned mango or diced fresh peaches, nectarines or papaya.
• As a variation, replace the flour tortillas with corn tortillas. This will also increase the fibre content a little.
• You can heat the tortillas in a 180°C (350°F/Gas 4) oven for 8 minutes, and cook the prawns in a chargrill pan or frying pan if you don't have a barbecue.

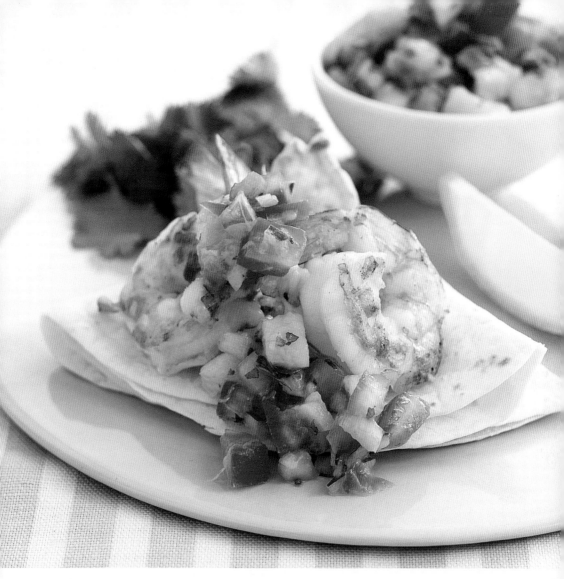

THESE TORTILLAS ARE QUICK AND
EASY TO MAKE AND ARE GREAT AS
A SNACK OR LIGHT MEAL. THE
SALSA IS AN EXCELLENT SOURCE
OF TWO MAJOR ANTIOXIDANTS—
BETA-CAROTENE AND VITAMIN C.

nutrition per tortilla: Energy 821 kJ (196 Cal)
Fat 3.1 g
Saturated fat 0.4 g
Protein 12.3 g
Carbohydrate 27.5 g
Fibre 3.3 g
Cholesterol 57 mg

SOUPS

BEEF AND CHILLI BEAN SOUP

THIS SOUP IS A HEARTY, LOW-GI MAIN MEAL IN A BOWL, AND IS A GOOD SOURCE OF IRON AND ZINC. MAKE THE SOUP A DAY AHEAD AND REFRIGERATE IT OVERNIGHT TO GIVE IT TIME TO DEVELOP ITS FULL FLAVOUR.

1 tbsp olive oil

1 red onion, finely chopped

2 garlic cloves, crushed

2½ tsp chilli flakes

2½ tsp ground cumin

1½ tsp ground coriander

2½ tbsp finely chopped coriander (cilantro) root and stem

500 g (1 lb 2 oz) lean minced (ground) beef

2 litres (70 fl oz/8 cups) beef stock

4 tomatoes, seeded and diced

1 tbsp tomato paste (concentrated purée)

420 g (15 oz) tin red kidney beans, drained and rinsed

3 tbsp chopped coriander (cilantro) leaves

90 g (3¼ oz/⅓ cup) light sour cream

PREP TIME: 20 MINUTES

COOKING TIME: 30 MINUTES

SERVES 4

Heat the oil in a large saucepan over medium heat and cook the onion for 2–3 minutes, or until softened. Add the garlic, chilli flakes, ground cumin, ground coriander and coriander root and stem and cook for another minute. Add the beef and cook for 3–4 minutes, or until cooked through, breaking up any lumps with the back of a wooden spoon.

Add the stock, tomatoes, tomato paste and kidney beans and bring to the boil over high heat. Reduce the heat and simmer for 15–20 minutes, or until reduced slightly. Remove any skum that rises to the surface. Stir in the coriander leaves and season with salt and freshly ground black pepper. Divide among four serving bowls and top with a dollop of sour cream.

nutrition per serve: Energy 1783 kJ (426 Cal); Fat 17 g; Saturated fat 5.9 g; Protein 41.2 g; Carbohydrate 22.5 g; Fibre 8 g; Cholesterol 77 mg

WINTER LAMB SHANK SOUP

BARLEY IS AN EXCELLENT SOURCE OF SOLUBLE FIBRE AND IS A VERY
FILLING FOOD, SO THIS HEARTY WINTER SOUP IS A GREAT CHOICE FOR
PEOPLE WHO ARE WATCHING THEIR WEIGHT.

1 tbsp olive oil

1.25 kg (2 lb 12 oz) trimmed lamb shanks

2 onions, chopped

4 garlic cloves, chopped

250 ml (9 fl oz/1 cup) red wine

2 bay leaves

1 tbsp chopped rosemary

2.5 litres (87 fl oz/10 cups) beef stock

400 g (14 oz) tin crushed tomatoes

165 g (5¾ oz/¾ cup) pearl barley, rinsed
 and drained

1 large carrot, unpeeled, diced

1 potato, unpeeled, diced

1 turnip, peeled and diced

1 parsnip, peeled and diced

2 tbsp redcurrant jelly (optional)

PREP TIME: 30 MINUTES

COOKING TIME: 4 HOURS

SERVES 6

Heat the oil in a large saucepan or stockpot over high heat. Add the shanks and cook for
2–3 minutes, or until browned. Remove and set aside.

Add the onion to the pan and cook over low heat for 8 minutes, or until softened. Add the
garlic and cook for a further 30 seconds, then add the wine and simmer for 5 minutes,
scraping up any sediment stuck to the bottom of the pan.

Return the shanks to the pan along with the bay leaves and half the rosemary. Pour in
1.5 litres (52 fl oz/6 cups) of the stock and season with salt and pepper. Bring to the boil
over high heat, then reduce the heat and simmer, covered, for 2 hours, or until the meat
is falling off the bones.

Remove the shanks and cool slightly. Remove the meat from the bones and roughly chop.
Add the meat to the broth along with the tomatoes, barley and remaining rosemary and
stock. Simmer for 30 minutes. Add the vegetables and cook for 1 hour, or until the barley
is tender. Remove the bay leaves and stir in the redcurrant jelly, if using. Serve immediately.

HINTS:
• This soup will thicken on standing. It may be necessary to thin the soup with extra stock
  or water when reheating.
• Freeze any leftover soup in an airtight container for up to 1 month.

nutrition per serve: Energy 1812 kJ (433 Cal); Fat 11.6 g; Saturated fat 4.1 g; Protein 36.2 g;
Carbohydrate 35.3 g; Fibre 6.6 g; Cholesterol 84 mg

LENTIL AND VEGETABLE SOUP WITH SPICED YOGHURT

2 tbsp olive oil

1 small leek, white part only, chopped

2 garlic cloves, crushed

2 tsp curry powder

1 tsp ground cumin

1 tsp garam masala

1 litre (35 fl oz/4 cups) vegetable stock

1 bay leaf

185 g (6½ oz/1 cup) brown lentils

450 g (1 lb) butternut pumpkin (squash),
    peeled and cut into 1 cm (½ in) cubes

2 zucchini (courgettes), cut in half
    lengthways and sliced

400 g (14 oz) tin chopped tomatoes

200 g (7 oz) broccoli, cut into small florets

1 small carrot, diced

80 g (2¾ oz/½ cup) peas

1 tbsp chopped mint

SPICED YOGHURT

250 g (9 oz/1 cup) Greek-style yoghurt

1 tbsp chopped coriander (cilantro) leaves

1 garlic clove, crushed

3 dashes Tabasco sauce

PREP TIME: 20 MINUTES

COOKING TIME: 35 MINUTES

SERVES 6

Heat the olive oil in a saucepan over medium heat, add the leek and garlic and cook for 4–5 minutes, or until soft and lightly golden. Add the curry powder, cumin and garam masala and cook for 1 minute, or until fragrant.

Add the stock, bay leaf, lentils and pumpkin. Bring to the boil, then reduce the heat to low and simmer for 10–15 minutes, or until the lentils are tender. Season well.

Add the zucchini, tomatoes, broccoli, carrot and 500 ml (17 fl oz/2 cups) water and simmer for 10 minutes, or until the vegetables are tender. Add the peas and simmer for a further 2–3 minutes.

To make the spiced yoghurt, put the yoghurt, coriander, garlic and Tabasco in a small bowl and stir until combined. Dollop a spoonful of the yoghurt on each serving of soup and garnish with the chopped mint.

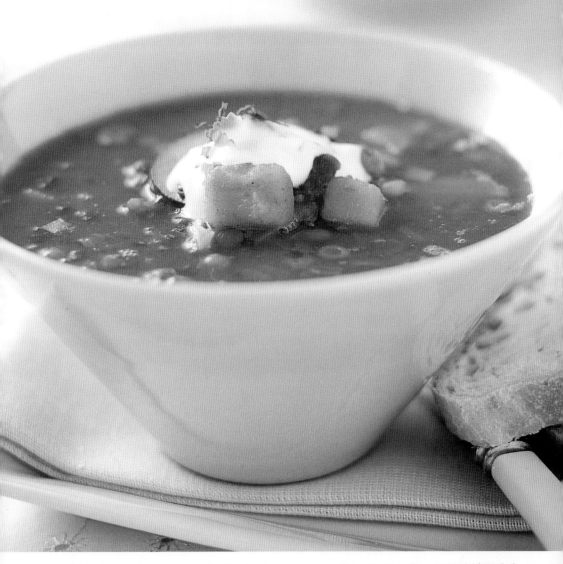

THIS COLOURFUL SOUP GIVES YOU THE FILLING POWER AND GOODNESS OF VEGETABLES AND LENTILS, AS WELL AS LOTS OF WONDERFUL AROMAS AND SPICY FLAVOURS. THIS SOUP IS AN EXCELLENT SOURCE OF THE ANTIOXIDANT, BETA-CAROTENE.

nutrition per serve: Energy 1140 kJ (272 Cal)
Fat 9.6 g
Saturated fat 2.3 g
Protein 15.2 g
Carbohydrate 26.9 g
Fibre 11.3 g
Cholesterol 20 mg

GAZPACHO

This chilled soup is an ideal meal for summer, when tomatoes are at their peak. For the best flavour, choose tomatoes that are fully ripe and red. Tomatoes are packed with the antioxidant, lycopene.

1 kg (2 lb 4 oz) vine-ripened tomatoes
½ telegraph (long) cucumber, roughly
   chopped
4 spring onions (scallions), thinly sliced
1 red capsicum (pepper), roughly chopped
2 garlic cloves, crushed
250 ml (9 fl oz/1 cup) chilled chicken stock
2 tbsp extra virgin olive oil
3 tbsp red wine vinegar
1 slice day-old Italian-style bread,
   roughly torn

1 small handful basil, shredded
40 g (1½ oz/⅓ cup) pitted black olives,
   sliced
4 wholegrain bread rolls, to serve

PREP TIME: 20 MINUTES
COOKING TIME: NIL
SERVES 4

To peel the tomatoes, score a cross in the base of each tomato. Put in a heatproof bowl and cover with boiling water. Leave for 30 seconds, then transfer to cold water and peel the skin away from the cross. Roughly cut into quarters.

Place the tomatoes in a large bowl and add the cucumber, spring onion, capsicum, garlic, stock, oil, vinegar and bread. Mix well.

Process the mixture in a blender or food processor in batches, taking care to add enough of the liquid so the mixture blends easily. Thin the soup with water or more stock if desired. Season to taste with salt and freshly ground black pepper and serve chilled, garnished with the basil and olives. Serve with the bread rolls.

nutrition per serve: Energy 1359 kJ (325 Cal); Fat 12 g; Saturated fat 1.6 g; Protein 10.3 g; Carbohydrate 39 g; Fibre 7.6 g; Cholesterol 0 mg

SPLIT PEA SOUP

A GREAT WAY TO INCLUDE LEGUMES IN YOUR DIET, THIS DELICIOUS SOUP
PROVIDES GOOD AMOUNTS OF SOLUBLE FIBRE, FOLATE AND BETA-CAROTENE.
USE GLUTEN-FREE STOCK FOR A GLUTEN-FREE MEAL.

2 tbsp olive oil
1 large onion, chopped
1 large carrot, cut into 1 cm (½ in) cubes
1 large celery stalk, cut into 1 cm (½ in)
    cubes
2 bay leaves
1 tbsp thyme, finely chopped
6 garlic cloves, finely chopped
440 g (15½ oz/2 cups) yellow split peas

1 litre (35 fl oz/4 cups) chicken stock
3 tbsp lemon juice
olive oil, extra, to serve

PREP TIME: 20 MINUTES
COOKING TIME: 1 HOUR 20 MINUTES
SERVES 6–8

Heat the oil in a large saucepan over medium heat. Add the onion, carrot and celery and cook for 4–5 minutes, or until starting to brown. Add the bay leaves, thyme and garlic and cook for 1 minute.

Stir in the split peas, then add the stock and 1 litre (35 fl oz/4 cups) water. Cook for 1 hour 15 minutes, or until the split peas and vegetables are soft. Stir often during cooking to prevent the soup from sticking to the bottom of the pan, and skim any scum from the surface. Add a little extra water if the soup is too thick.

Remove from the heat and discard the bay leaves. Stir in the lemon juice and season with salt and freshly ground black pepper. Drizzle with a little olive oil before serving.

nutrition per serve (8): Energy 998 kJ (239 Cal); Fat 6.1 g; Saturated fat 0.8 g; Protein 14.7 g; Carbohydrate 28.4 g; Fibre 6.5 g; Cholesterol 0 mg

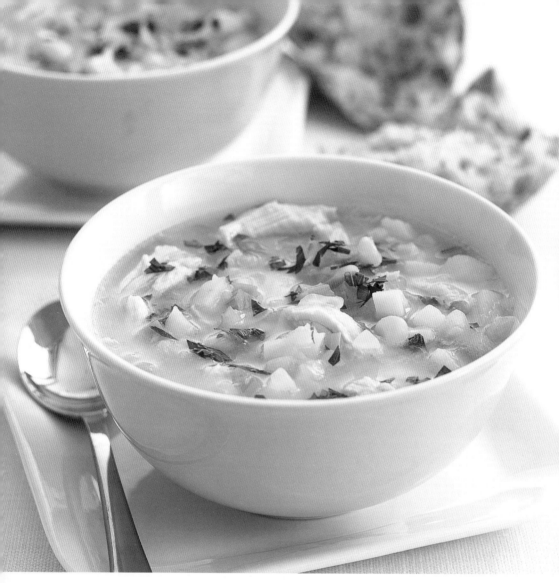

MAKE A FILLING AND NUTRITIOUS
MEAL OF THIS DELICIOUS
CHOWDER BY SERVING IT WITH
CRUSTY WHOLEGRAIN BREAD AND
SALAD. THIS IS A THICK SOUP, SO
ADD MORE STOCK OR MILK TO THIN
IT, IF DESIRED.

nutrition per serve: Energy 1285 kJ (307 Cal)

Fat 2.3 g

Saturated fat 0.6 g

Protein 21.4 g

Carbohydrate 45.5 g

Fibre 8.1 g

Cholesterol 33 mg

CHICKEN CORN CHOWDER

180 g (6 oz) boneless skinless chicken
   breast, trimmed
1 litre (35 fl oz/4 cups) chicken stock
   or water
1 large onion, diced
2 potatoes, diced
1 celery stalk, diced
1 large carrot, grated
420 g (15 oz) tin creamed corn

310 g (11 oz) tin corn kernels, drained and
   rinsed
125 ml (4 fl oz/½ cup) skim or no-fat milk
3 tbsp finely chopped flat-leaf (Italian)
   parsley

PREP TIME: 15 MINUTES
COOKING TIME: 35 MINUTES
SERVES 4

Cut 2–3 slits across the thickest part of the chicken. Heat the stock in a large heavy-based saucepan, add the chicken and poach for 10 minutes, or until just cooked through. Remove the chicken from the pan and set aside. When cooled, use two forks to thinly shred the chicken flesh.

Add the onion, potato, celery and carrot to the saucepan. Bring to the boil, then lower the heat and simmer for 20 minutes, or until the potato is cooked.

Stir in the chicken, creamed corn, corn kernels, milk and parsley. Stir gently to heat through and serve.

HINTS:
• Instead of poaching the chicken, use the skinless fat-free breast meat from a barbecued chicken. Frozen precooked chicken breasts are also available in the freezer section of the supermarket.
• This soup is best eaten on the day it is made, although you can freeze the soup into serving-sized portions.

ROASTED VEGETABLE SOUP

THE MORE YOU PROCESS OR CHOP UP FIBRE, THE LESS EFFECTIVE IT WILL
BE IN YOUR BODY. THE VEGETABLES IN THIS RUSTIC SOUP HAVE ONLY BEEN
ROUGHLY MASHED INSTEAD OF PURÉED IN A BLENDER.

750 g (1 lb 10 oz) unpeeled carrots,
chopped into 5 cm (2 in) pieces
350 g (12 oz) unpeeled orange sweet
potato, chopped into 5 cm (2 in) pieces
2 zucchini (courgettes), halved lengthways
1 tbsp olive oil
2 onions, cut into wedges
3 unpeeled garlic cloves
1 bay leaf
4 parsley stalks

2 thyme sprigs
1.5 litres (52 fl oz/6 cups) chicken stock
400 g (14 oz) tin chopped tomatoes
1 tbsp tomato paste (concentrated purée)
4 thin slices pancetta or prosciutto,
chopped

PREP TIME: 20 MINUTES
COOKING TIME: 1½ HOURS
SERVES 4–6

Preheat the oven to 180°C (350°F/Gas 4). Put the carrot, sweet potato and zucchini in
a large shallow roasting tin. Drizzle with the oil and toss to coat the vegetables. Bake for
30 minutes, then add the onion and garlic. Bake for a further 30 minutes, or until the
vegetables are tender and lightly browned. Turn the vegetables occasionally during baking.
Peel the garlic cloves.

Transfer the garlic and the contents of the roasting tin to a large saucepan. Tie the bay leaf,
parsley stalks and thyme sprigs together and add to the pan. Add the stock, tomatoes and
tomato paste. Bring to the boil, then reduce the heat and simmer for 20 minutes. Cool for
10 minutes, then remove the bay leaf, parsley and thyme sprigs. Use a potato masher to
roughly mash the vegetables. Season with salt and freshly ground black pepper.

Heat a small frying pan over medium heat, add the pancetta and cook until crisp. Reheat
the soup just before serving and sprinkle over the crumbled pancetta. Serve with crunchy
wholegrain bread or toast.

HINTS:
• Make a vegetarian version of this soup by using vegetable stock or water and omitting
the pancetta or prosciutto.
• Freeze any leftover soup in an airtight container for up to 1 month.

nutrition per serve (6): Energy 757 kJ (181 Cal); Fat 4.6 g; Saturated fat 0.8 g; Protein 8.6 g;
Carbohydrate 23 g; Fibre 7 g; Cholesterol 3 mg

MEDITERRANEAN FISH SOUP

THIS DELICIOUS SOUP EVOKES THE WARMTH OF THE MEDITERRANEAN AND IS A GREAT WAY TO INCLUDE FISH IN YOUR DIET. IT'S LOW IN FAT AND CONTAINS PROTEIN, ANTIOXIDANTS AND B-GROUP VITAMINS.

½ tsp saffron threads

2 tsp olive oil

1 large onion, thinly sliced

1 leek, white part only, chopped

4 garlic cloves, finely chopped

½ tsp dried oregano

1 tsp grated orange zest

2 tbsp dry white wine

1 red capsicum (pepper), cut into bite-sized pieces

2 zucchini (courgettes), chopped

500 g (1 lb 2 oz) ripe tomatoes, chopped

125 ml (4 fl oz/½ cup) tomato passata (puréed tomatoes)

750 ml (26 fl oz/3 cups) fish stock

2 tbsp tomato paste (concentrated purée)

2 tsp soft brown sugar

500 g (1 lb 2 oz) skinless and boneless fish fillets, trimmed and cut into bite-sized pieces

300 g (10½ oz) tin red kidney beans, drained and rinsed

4 tbsp chopped parsley

4 wholegrain bread rolls

PREP TIME: 30 MINUTES

COOKING TIME: 45 MINUTES

SERVES 4

Soak the saffron threads in a small bowl with 2 tablespoons boiling water.

Heat the oil in a large saucepan over low heat. Add the onion, leek, garlic and oregano. Cover and cook for 10 minutes, shaking the pan occasionally, until the onion is soft. Add the orange zest, wine, capsicum, zucchini and tomatoes, cover and cook for 10 minutes.

Add the tomato passata, stock, tomato paste, sugar and saffron (along with the soaking water) to the pan. Stir well and bring to the boil, then reduce the heat to low and simmer, uncovered, for 15 minutes.

Add the fish to the soup, cover and cook for 8 minutes, or until tender. Add the kidney beans and half the parsley and season to taste with salt and freshly ground black pepper. Sprinkle the soup with the remaining parsley just before serving. Serve with bread rolls.

HINTS:
• Try fish such as snapper, red mullet, red rock cod or ocean perch.
• Passata, or Italian tomato purée, is available in jars at supermarkets.

nutrition per serve: Energy 1827 kJ (436 Cal); Fat 6.9 g; Saturated fat 1.2 g; Protein 38.4 g; Carbohydrate 47 g; Fibre 11.8 g; Cholesterol 51 mg

HEARTY BEAN AND VEGETABLE SOUP

1 tsp olive oil
100 g (3½ oz) pancetta, trimmed and diced
1 leek, white part only, thinly sliced
2 garlic cloves, chopped
1 celery stalk, thinly sliced
1 large carrot, diced
2 waxy potatoes, diced
2 litres (70 fl oz/8 cups) chicken stock
400 g (14 oz) tin chopped tomatoes
80 g (2¾ oz/½ cup) macaroni
155 g (5½ oz/1 cup) frozen peas, thawed
1 zucchini (courgette), thinly sliced

185 g (6½ oz) cauliflower, cut into small
 florets
400 g (14 oz) tin cannellini beans, drained
 and rinsed
1 handful flat-leaf (Italian) parsley, chopped
grated parmesan cheese, to serve
 (optional)

PREP TIME: 25 MINUTES

COOKING TIME: 40 MINUTES

SERVES 4–6

Heat the oil in a large saucepan over low heat. Add the pancetta, leek and garlic and cook, stirring, for 10 minutes, without browning. Add the celery, carrot and potato. Cook for a further 5 minutes, stirring.

Pour in the stock and add the tomatoes. Bring slowly to the boil, then reduce the heat and simmer for 15 minutes. Stir in the pasta, peas, zucchini, cauliflower and cannellini beans. Simmer for a further 10 minutes, or until the pasta is cooked.

Before serving, stir in the parsley. Serve with grated parmesan if desired, and crusty wholegrain bread.

HINTS:
• As a variation, you can use red kidney beans instead of cannellini beans.
• If pancetta is not available, use 97% fat-free bacon.
• Freeze any leftover soup into serving-sized portions. It will keep for up to 1 month.

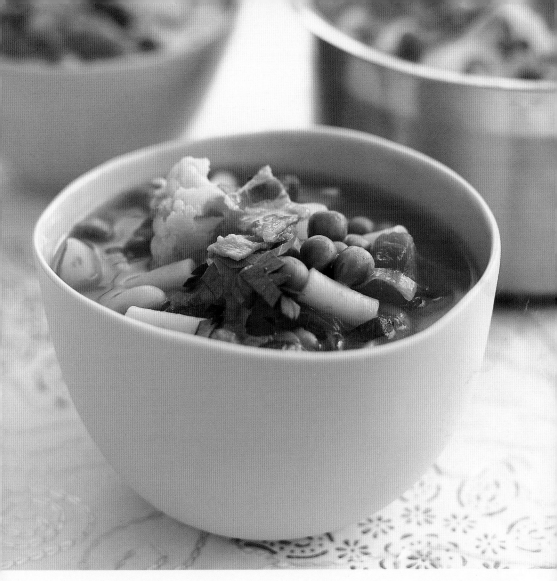

IT ISN'T DIFFICULT TO EAT A
VARIETY OF HEALTHY FOODS,
AND WITH THIS VEGETABLE
SOUP YOU CAN DO THAT IN ONE
MEAL. FULL OF GOODNESS AND
WONDERFUL FLAVOURS, THIS
VITAMIN-RICH SOUP HITS THE
SPOT EVERY TIME.

nutrition per serve (6): Energy 1060 kJ (253 Cal)
Fat 4.2 g
Saturated fat 1.2 g
Protein 17.6 g
Carbohydrate 32.4 g
Fibre 8.5 g
Cholesterol 16 mg

97

PEA AND HAM SOUP

This nourishing soup is a great way to include more legumes in your diet. Using sweet potato instead of regular potato reduces the GI of the soup—a better choice for those with diabetes.

440 g (15½ oz/2 cups) split green peas, rinsed and drained
750 g (1 lb 10 oz) ham bones
1 celery stalk, including leaves, chopped
1 carrot, diced
1 onion, chopped
3 leeks, sliced
1 orange sweet potato, peeled and chopped

Prep time: 20 minutes + 4 hours soaking
Cooking time: 2½ hours
Serves 4–6

Put the split peas in a large bowl, cover with water and leave to soak for at least 4 hours or overnight. Drain and rinse well.

Put the ham bones, split peas, celery, carrot and onion in a large saucepan with 2.5 litres (87 fl oz/10 cups) water. Bring to the boil, then reduce the heat and simmer, covered, for 2 hours, or until the split peas are very soft.

Add the leek and sweet potato to the pan and cook for 30 minutes, or until the vegetables are tender and the ham is falling off the bone. Remove the ham bones from the soup, cut off all the meat and finely chop.

Transfer the soup to a bowl to cool, then use a potato masher to lightly mash—the soup should be chunky. Return the soup to the pan, stir in the chopped ham and reheat the soup to serve. Either serve the soup on its own as a starter, or serve with toasted wholegrain bread and salad as a complete meal.

HINT:
• Some ham can be quite salty—soaking the bone in cold water overnight will draw out a lot of the saltiness.

nutrition per serve (6): Energy 1564 kJ (374 Cal); Fat 7.1 g; Saturated fat 2.2 g; Protein 31.7 g; Carbohydrate 41.4 g; Fibre 9.8 g; Cholesterol 32 mg

RED LENTIL, BURGHUL AND MINT SOUP

THIS LOW-GI SOUP IS A RICH SOURCE OF FIBRE AND HAS GOOD AMOUNTS OF FOLATE AND BETA-CAROTENE. FOR A VEGETARIAN MEAL, REPLACE THE CHICKEN STOCK WITH VEGETABLE STOCK.

2 tomatoes, finely chopped
2 tbsp olive oil
1 large red onion, finely chopped
2 garlic cloves, crushed
2 tbsp tomato paste (concentrated purée)
2 tsp ground paprika
½ tsp cayenne pepper
400 g (14 oz/2 cups) red lentils
50 g (1¾ oz/¼ cup) basmati rice
2.125 litres (74 fl oz/8½ cups) chicken stock

50 g (1¾ oz/¼ cup) fine burghul (bulgur)
2 tbsp chopped mint
2 tbsp chopped flat-leaf (Italian) parsley
90 g (3¼ oz/⅓ cup) low-fat plain yoghurt
¼ preserved lemon, pulp removed, rind washed and cut into thin strips

PREP TIME: 25 MINUTES
COOKING TIME: 45 MINUTES
SERVES 4–6

To peel the tomatoes, score a cross in the base of each tomato. Put in a heatproof bowl and cover with boiling water. Leave for 30 seconds, then transfer to cold water and peel the skin away from the cross. Finely chop the flesh.

Heat the oil in a large saucepan over medium heat. Add the onion and garlic and cook for 2–3 minutes, or until soft. Stir in the tomatoes, tomato paste, paprika and cayenne pepper and cook for 1 minute.

Add the lentils, rice and stock, cover and bring to the boil over high heat. Reduce the heat and simmer for 30–35 minutes, or until the rice is cooked.

Stir in the burghul, mint and parsley and season with salt and freshly ground black pepper. Divide the soup among serving bowls and garnish with the yoghurt and preserved lemon. Serve immediately.

HINT:
• This soup will thicken on standing, so if reheating you may need to add more liquid.

nutrition per serve (6): Energy 1554 kJ (371 Cal); Fat 8.2 g; Saturated fat 1.3 g; Protein 24.7 g; Carbohydrate 44.5 g; Fibre 12.5 g; Cholesterol 1 mg

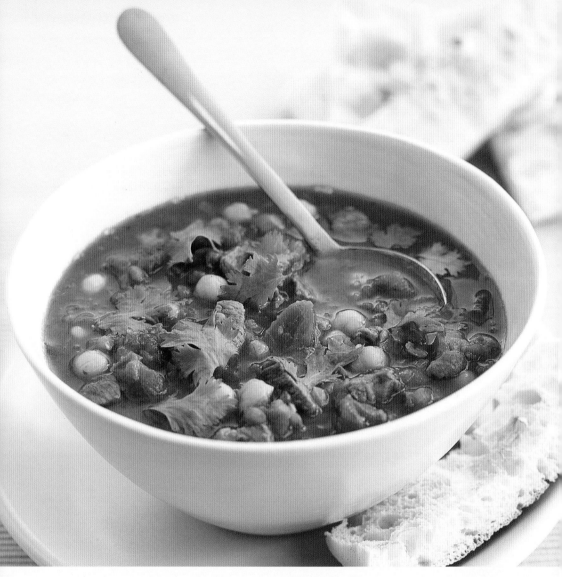

THIS FLAVOURSOME, HEARTY HIGH-FIBRE SOUP IS HIGH IN PROTEIN AND CONTAINS GOOD AMOUNTS OF IRON AND ZINC. TOMATOES ARE A RICH SOURCE OF THE ANTIOXIDANT, LYCOPENE.

nutrition per serve (6): Energy 1877 kJ (448 Cal)
Fat 14.2 g
Saturated fat 4.9 g
Protein 45.8 g
Carbohydrate 28 g
Fibre 10.1 g
Cholesterol 96 mg

MOROCCAN CHICKPEA, LAMB AND CORIANDER SOUP

165 g (5¾ oz/¾ cup) dried chickpeas
1 tbsp olive oil
850 g (1 lb 14 oz) boned lamb leg, cut into
   1 cm (½ in) cubes
1 onion, chopped
2 garlic cloves, crushed
½ tsp ground cinnamon
½ tsp ground turmeric
½ tsp ground ginger
4 tbsp chopped coriander (cilantro) leaves

2 x 400 g (14 oz) tins diced tomatoes
1 litre (35 fl oz/4 cups) chicken stock
135 g (4¾ oz/⅔ cup) red lentils
fresh coriander (cilantro) leaves, to garnish
Turkish bread, to serve

PREP TIME: 15 MINUTES + OVERNIGHT
   SOAKING
COOKING TIME: 2¼ HOURS
SERVES 4–6

Put the chickpeas in a large bowl, cover with water and soak overnight. Drain and rinse under cold water and drain again.

Heat the oil in a large saucepan over high heat. Add the lamb and brown in batches for 2–3 minutes. Reduce the heat to medium, return all the lamb to the pan along with the onion and garlic and cook for 5 minutes. Add the cinnamon, turmeric, ginger, a pinch of salt and 1 teaspoon freshly ground black pepper and cook for a further 2 minutes. Add the chopped coriander, tomatoes, stock and 500 ml (17 fl oz/2 cups) water and bring to the boil over high heat.

Rinse the lentils under cold water and drain. Add the lentils and chickpeas to the pan, then reduce the heat and simmer, covered, for 1½ hours. Uncover and cook for a further 30 minutes, or until the lamb is tender and the soup is thick. Season to taste. Divide the soup among serving bowls and garnish with the coriander leaves. Serve with toasted Turkish bread.

MAIN MEALS

CHICKEN AND NOODLE STIR-FRY

HIGH IN PROTEIN AND LOW IN FAT, THIS IS A QUICK AND EASY WEEKNIGHT STIR-FRY. REPLACE THE DRIED NOODLES WITH FRESH RICE NOODLES FOR A LOWER GI MEAL.

200 g (7 oz) dried rice noodles
3 tbsp chopped fresh ginger
2 garlic cloves, finely chopped
1 tsp sesame oil
200 g (7 oz) broccolini, cut into 5 cm
    (2 in) pieces
1 large red capsicum (pepper), thinly sliced
100 g (3½ oz) snowpeas (mangetout)
    or sugar snap peas, thinly sliced on
    the diagonal
4 spring onions (scallions), sliced
2 tsp olive oil
500 g (1 lb 2 oz) boneless skinless chicken
    breasts, cut into strips

1 tbsp black bean sauce
1 tbsp oyster sauce or soy sauce
1 tbsp hoisin sauce
1 tbsp chilli sauce or ½ large chilli,
    finely chopped
80 ml (2½ fl oz/⅓ cup) chicken stock
    or water
4 tbsp roughly chopped coriander
    (cilantro) leaves and stalks

PREP TIME: 20 MINUTES + 10 MINUTES
    SOAKING
COOKING TIME: 10 MINUTES
SERVES 4

Soak the rice noodles in hot water, immersing them completely. Mix well to break up the noodles and prevent them sticking together. Leave to soften for 10 minutes, then drain.

Meanwhile, put the ginger and garlic in a wok. Pour the sesame oil over the top and turn the heat to high. Cook for about 1 minute, or until the wok is hot. Add the vegetables and cook for 2 minutes, stirring frequently, until tender. Transfer the vegetables to a bowl.

Heat the olive oil in the wok, add the chicken strips and stir-fry for 2 minutes, or until just cooked. Add the black bean sauce, oyster sauce, hoisin sauce and chilli sauce. Stir to combine, then transfer the chicken to the bowl with the vegetables, leaving behind as much liquid as possible in the wok.

Add the drained noodles and stock to the wok and cook for 1–2 minutes, or until the noodles are soft. Return the chicken and vegetables to the wok along with the coriander. Remove from the heat and stir until well mixed. Serve immediately.

nutrition per serve: Energy 1611 kJ (385 Cal); Fat 6.8 g; Saturated fat 1.4 g; Protein 35.3 g; Carbohydrate 42.1 g; Fibre 5.3 g; Cholesterol 87 mg

LAMB SOUVLAKI

FOR COLOUR AND VARIETY, ADD SOME ONION AND GREEN CAPSICUM (PEPPER) PIECES TO THESE DELICIOUS GREEK LAMB SKEWERS. YOU WILL NEED TO START THIS RECIPE A DAY AHEAD SO THE LAMB HAS TIME TO MARINATE.

2 tsp olive oil

2 tsp finely grated lemon zest

80 ml (2½ fl oz/⅓ cup) lemon juice

2 tsp dried oregano

125 ml (4 fl oz/½ cup) dry white wine

3 garlic cloves, finely chopped

2 fresh bay leaves

1 kg (2 lb 4 oz) boned leg lamb

250 g (9 oz/1 cup) low-fat plain yoghurt

2 garlic cloves, crushed, extra

olive oil spray

4 wholemeal (whole-wheat) pitta breads, to serve

PREP TIME: 20 MINUTES + OVERNIGHT MARINATING

COOKING TIME: 10 MINUTES

SERVES 4

To make the marinade, combine the oil, lemon zest, lemon juice, oregano, wine, garlic and bay leaves in a large non-metallic bowl. Season with salt and freshly ground black pepper. Trim the lamb and cut into bite-sized cubes. Add to the marinade and toss to coat well. Cover and refrigerate overnight.

Put the yoghurt and extra garlic in a bowl, mix together well and leave for 30 minutes. If using wooden skewers, soak them in cold water for about 30 minutes, to prevent the skewers burning during cooking.

Drain the lamb and pat dry. Thread the lamb onto eight metal or wooden skewers. Spray the barbecue hotplate with oil and heat to high. Add the lamb skewers and cook, turning them frequently, for 7–8 minutes, or until evenly brown on the outside and still a little rare in the middle.

Meanwhile, wrap the pitta breads in foil and put in a warm place on the barbecue for 10 minutes to heat through. Drizzle the lamb skewers with the garlic yoghurt and serve on the warm pitta bread with a green salad.

nutrition per serve: Energy 2686 kJ (642 Cal); Fat 19.4 g; Saturated fat 8 g; Protein 65.3 g; Carbohydrate 41.6 g; Fibre 6 g; Cholesterol 173 mg

PORK AND CHICKPEA STEW

2 tsp ground cumin

1 tsp ground coriander

½ tsp chilli powder

¼ tsp ground cinnamon

400 g (14 oz) lean diced pork, trimmed

1 tbsp plain (all-purpose) flour

1 tbsp olive oil

1 large onion, finely chopped

3 garlic cloves, finely chopped

2 large unpeeled carrots, chopped

2 celery stalks, sliced

250 ml (9 fl oz/1 cup) chicken stock

2 ripe tomatoes, chopped

310 g (11 oz) tin chickpeas, drained and
 rinsed

2 tbsp chopped parsley

PREP TIME: 30 MINUTES

COOKING TIME: 1½ HOURS

SERVES 4

Cook the spices in a dry frying pan over low heat, shaking the pan, for 1 minute, or until the spices are fragrant.

Combine the trimmed pork with the spices and flour in a plastic bag and toss well to coat. Remove the pork from the bag and shake off the excess flour.

Heat the oil in a large heavy-based saucepan over high heat and cook the pork, tossing regularly, for 8 minutes, or until lightly browned. Add the onion, garlic, carrot, celery and half the stock to the pan and toss well. Cover and cook for 10 minutes.

Add the remaining stock and tomato and season with salt and freshly ground black pepper. Bring to the boil, reduce the heat and cover with a tight-fitting lid, then simmer over low heat for 1 hour. Gently shake the pan occasionally but don't remove the lid during cooking. Stir in the chickpeas and parsley. Simmer, uncovered, for a further 5 minutes and serve.

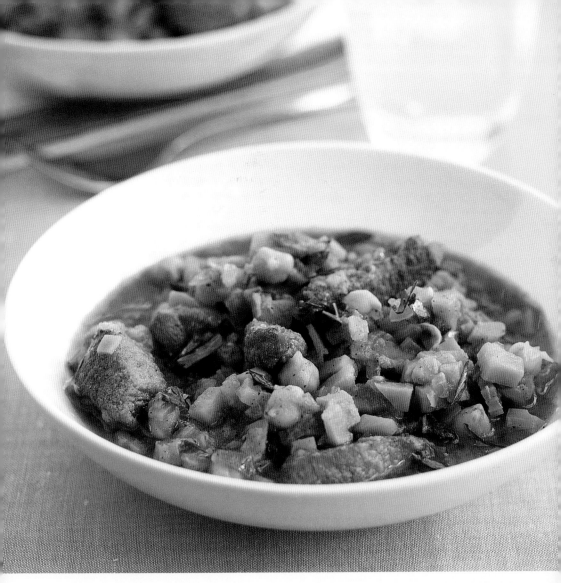

FOR A HEARTY WINTER STEW, YOU CAN'T BEAT THIS TASTY COMBINATION OF MEAT AND CHICKPEAS. PLUS, YOU'RE GETTING LOTS OF PROTEIN, SOME B-GROUP VITAMINS AND BETA-CAROTENE.

nutrition per serve: Energy 1128 kJ (269 Cal)
Fat 8.6 g
Saturated fat 1.7 g
Protein 28.5 g
Carbohydrate 16.5 g
Fibre 6.5 g
Cholesterol 95 mg

107

CHICKEN, CANNELLINI BEAN AND ZUCCHINI STEW

YOU CAN MAKE THIS RECIPE ON THE WEEKEND AND FREEZE IT IN INDIVIDUAL PORTIONS, WHICH CAN THEN BE THAWED AND REHEATED FOR A QUICK WEEKDAY MEAL.

2 tsp olive oil
8 boneless skinless chicken thighs,
  trimmed
1 onion, thinly sliced
4 garlic cloves, finely chopped
3 tbsp white wine
250 ml (9 fl oz/1 cup) chicken stock
1 tbsp finely chopped rosemary
1 tsp grated lemon zest
1 bay leaf

2 x 400 g (14 oz) tins cannellini beans,
  drained and rinsed
3 zucchini (courgettes), halved lengthways,
  then sliced on the diagonal
375 g (13 oz) fusilli

PREP TIME: 20 MINUTES

COOKING TIME: 1 HOUR 10 MINUTES

SERVES 4–6

Heat the oil in a large flameproof casserole dish. Add the chicken in batches and cook over medium heat for 4 minutes on each side, or until browned. Remove the chicken from the dish. Add the onion and cook for 5 minutes, or until softened. Add the garlic and cook for 1 minute, or until fragrant, then pour in the wine and stock and bring to the boil, scraping the bottom of the dish to remove any sediment.

Return the chicken and any juices to the dish along with the rosemary, lemon zest and bay leaf. Reduce the heat to low and simmer, covered, for 40 minutes, or until the chicken is tender. Stir in the cannellini beans and zucchini and cook for a further 5 minutes, or until the zucchini is tender.

Meanwhile, cook the pasta in a large saucepan of boiling water for 10 minutes, or until *al dente*. Drain and serve with the chicken. Serve with a mixed leaf salad dressed with oil and vinegar.

HINTS:
• To reduce the fat content, use boneless skinless chicken breasts, as these have less fat than thighs.
• As a variation, serve the stew with crusty wholegrain bread instead of pasta.

nutrition per serve (6): Energy 2369 kJ (566 Cal); Fat 17.7 g; Saturated fat 5.5 g; Protein 39.2 g; Carbohydrate 56.9 g; Fibre 9.3 g; Cholesterol 111 mg

CHILLI CON CARNE WITH PARSLEY RICE

THIS POPULAR DISH IS LOW GI AND IS GREAT FOR A FAMILY MEAL OR CASUAL DINNER PARTY. TO SAVE TIME, YOU CAN COOK THE CHILLI BEEF AHEAD OF TIME AND STORE IT IN THE REFRIGERATOR FOR UP TO 3 DAYS.

2 tsp olive oil
1 onion, chopped
3 garlic cloves, crushed
1 celery stalk, sliced
500 g (1 lb 2 oz) lean minced (ground) beef
2 tsp chilli powder
pinch of cayenne pepper
1 tbsp chopped oregano
400 g (14 oz) tin chopped tomatoes
2 tbsp tomato paste (concentrated purée)
300 g (10½ oz/1½ cups) basmati rice, rinsed and drained

4 tbsp finely chopped parsley
1 tsp soft brown sugar
1 tbsp cider vinegar or red wine vinegar
400 g (14 oz) tin red kidney beans, drained and rinsed
plain yoghurt or grated low-fat cheddar cheese, to serve

PREP TIME: 15 MINUTES
COOKING TIME: 1 HOUR 10 MINUTES
SERVES 4

Heat the oil in a large heavy-based saucepan. Add the onion, garlic and celery and stir over medium heat for 5 minutes, or until softened. Add the beef and cook over high heat for 5 minutes, or until well browned. Add the chilli powder, cayenne pepper and oregano. Stir well and cook for a further 5 minutes.

Add the tomatoes, tomato paste and 125 ml (4 fl oz/½ cup) water, stir well, then simmer for 30 minutes, stirring occasionally.

Meanwhile, put the rice and 750 ml (26 fl oz/3 cups) water in a saucepan and bring to the boil over medium heat. Reduce the heat to low, cover and cook for 20 minutes, or until the rice is tender. Remove from the heat and leave to stand, covered, for 5 minutes.

Add the parsley, sugar, vinegar and beans to the chilli mixture and season with salt and freshly ground black pepper. Heat through for 5 minutes before serving. Serve with the rice and top with a little yoghurt or cheese, if you like.

HINT:
• To increase the fibre content further, use a mixture of brown and white basmati rice.

nutrition per serve: Energy 2418 kJ (578 Cal); Fat 12.2 g; Saturated fat 4.1 g; Protein 36.3 g; Carbohydrate 75.5 g; Fibre 7.8 g; Cholesterol 64 mg

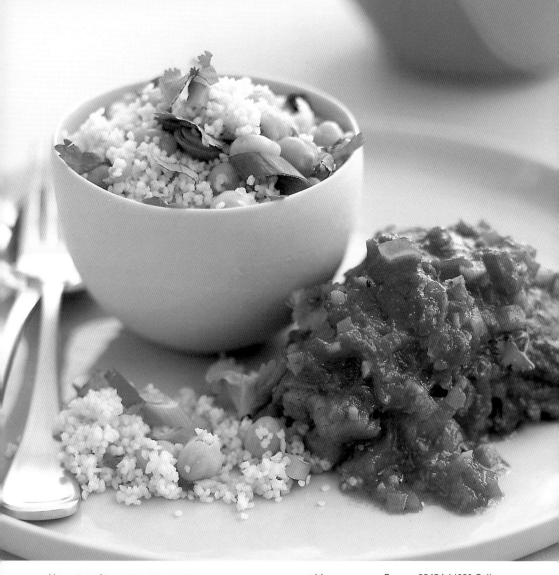

YOU DON'T NEED TO GO TO A
RESTAURANT FOR TASTY, EXOTIC
FOOD. THIS AROMATIC AFRICAN
MEAL CONTAINS ANTIOXIDANTS,
IRON AND B-GROUP VITAMINS,
INCLUDING FOLATE.

nutrition per serve: Energy 2845 kJ (680 Cal)
Fat 17.5 g
Saturated fat 4.3 g
Protein 55.4 g
Carbohydrate 70.5 g
Fibre 6.5 g
Cholesterol 170 mg

MOROCCAN CHICKEN ON COUSCOUS

1 tsp cumin seeds
1 tsp coriander seeds
1 tsp ground ginger
1 tsp ground turmeric
1 tsp ground cinnamon
½ tsp chilli flakes
8 skinless chicken pieces
3 tsp olive oil
1 onion, finely chopped
3 garlic cloves, crushed
1 tsp finely grated fresh ginger
400 g (14 oz) tin chopped tomatoes
250 ml (9 fl oz/1 cup) chicken stock

COUSCOUS
375 ml (13 fl oz/1½ cups) chicken stock
1 garlic clove, crushed
280 g (10 oz/1½ cups) couscous
400 g (14 oz) tin chickpeas
3 spring onions (scallions), thinly sliced on
   the diagonal
3 tbsp chopped coriander (cilantro) leaves

PREP TIME: 20 MINUTES + 15 MINUTES
   STANDING
COOKING TIME: 1 HOUR
SERVES 4

Put the cumin seeds, coriander seeds, ground ginger, turmeric, cinnamon and chilli flakes in a small heavy-based frying pan. Cook, stirring, over medium heat for 1 minute, or until fragrant. Grind the spices using a mortar and pestle or spice grinder to make a powder.

Sprinkle the chicken pieces with the spice mixture, rubbing in well. Heat 2 teaspoons of the oil in a large, deep heavy-based frying pan. Add the chicken and cook for 8 minutes, turning the pieces to brown evenly. Remove from the pan and set aside.

Add the remaining oil to the pan and cook the onion, garlic and ginger over medium heat for 3 minutes, or until softened. Add the tomatoes, stock and chicken to the pan. Bring to the boil, reduce the heat to low, cover and simmer for 45 minutes, or until the chicken is tender and the sauce has reduced. Season to taste.

Meanwhile, make the couscous. Put the stock and garlic in a small saucepan and bring to the boil. Put the couscous in a bowl and pour over the hot stock. Cover with plastic wrap and set aside for 15 minutes. Stir the couscous with a fork to fluff up the grains, then add the rinsed and drained chickpeas, spring onion and half the coriander. Season well. Serve the couscous with the Moroccan chicken. Sprinkle with the remaining coriander.

HINT:
• We used skinless chicken thighs with the bone, plus drumsticks. To reduce the amount of fat in the meal, use chicken drumsticks, as these have less fat than chicken thighs.

TUNA WITH CHICKPEAS AND ROAST TOMATO SALAD

TUNA IS A GOOD SOURCE OF ESSENTIAL OMEGA-3 FATTY ACIDS, WHICH MOST PEOPLE DON'T REGULARLY INCLUDE IN THEIR DIET. THIS DISH IS ALSO A GOOD SOURCE OF ZINC, IODINE AND SELENIUM.

220 g (7¾ oz/1 cup) dried chickpeas
6 roma (plum) tomatoes, cut into quarters
    lengthways
2 tbsp olive oil
4 x 150 g (5½ oz) tuna steaks
2 tbsp lemon juice
1 red onion, chopped
1 garlic clove, crushed
1 tsp ground cumin

2 large handfuls flat-leaf (Italian) parsley,
    roughly chopped
extra parsley, to garnish

PREP TIME: 10 MINUTES + OVERNIGHT
    SOAKING + 30 MINUTES MARINATING
COOKING TIME: 1 HOUR 25 MINUTES
SERVES 4

Soak the chickpeas in enough water to cover for 8 hours, or overnight. Drain and discard the liquid. Put the chickpeas in a saucepan with enough water to cover them and bring to the boil. Cook for 25–30 minutes, or until tender. Drain, then rinse well under cold water.

Preheat the oven to 180°C (350°F/Gas 4). Combine the tomatoes, 2 teaspoons of the olive oil, salt and freshly ground black pepper. Place the tomatoes on a baking tray and bake for 35–40 minutes, or until golden.

Brush the tuna steaks with 2 teaspoons of the olive oil and 1 tablespoon of the lemon juice. Season and place in the refrigerator to marinate for 30 minutes.

Heat the remaining olive oil in a frying pan over medium heat. Add the onion and garlic and cook, stirring, for 4–5 minutes, or until softened. Add the cumin and cook for a further minute, then add the chickpeas. Cook for 5 minutes, stirring occasionally. Add the roasted tomatoes, parsley and remaining lemon juice and gently stir to combine. Season with salt and freshly ground black pepper.

Heat a chargrill pan or barbecue chargrill plate to high. Add the tuna and cook on each side for 1–2 minutes, or until cooked to your liking. Serve the tuna on top of the warm chickpea salad and garnish with extra parsley.

nutrition per serve: Energy 2026 kJ (484 Cal); Fat 20.4 g; Saturated fat 5.1 g; Protein 47.8 g; Carbohydrate 21.4 g; Fibre 8.2 g; Cholesterol 54 mg

LEMON ROASTED CHICKEN WITH ROAST VEGETABLES

LEAVING THE SKINS ON THE GARLIC AND FRENCH SHALLOTS PREVENTS THEM FROM BURNING DURING COOKING. TO LOWER THE FAT AND CHOLESTEROL CONTENT OF THE MEAL, TAKE THE SKIN OFF THE CHICKEN BEFORE EATING IT.

1.4 kg (3 lb 2 oz) chicken

2 bay leaves

2 lemons

2 lemon thyme sprigs

2 marjoram sprigs

1 tbsp chopped lemon thyme

1 tbsp chopped marjoram

1 tbsp olive oil

12 baby new potatoes, unpeeled

300 g (10½ oz) orange sweet potato, peeled and cut into 8 pieces

8 French shallots, unpeeled

2 large zucchini (courgettes), halved lengthways, then halved again widthways

8 garlic cloves, unpeeled

PREP TIME: 20 MINUTES

COOKING TIME: 1 HOUR 10 MINUTES
+ 5 MINUTES RESTING

SERVES 4

Preheat the oven to 200°C (400°F/Gas 6). Pat the chicken dry with paper towels and place on a rack in a deep roasting tin. Season the cavity and put the bay leaves, 1 whole lemon and the lemon thyme and marjoram sprigs inside. Cut the remaining lemon in half and rub all over the chicken, then cut the lemon into quarters and reserve.

Season lightly and roast the chicken, basting every 20 minutes with the tin juices, for 1 hour 10 minutes, or until browned and the juices run clear when pierced between the thigh and the body. Remove the chicken from the rack and sit, covered lightly with foil, for 5 minutes.

Meanwhile, to roast the vegetables, combine the chopped lemon thyme and marjoram with the oil, salt, freshly ground black pepper and the reserved lemon quarters in a large bowl. Add all the vegetables and the unpeeled garlic cloves and toss together.

Put the potatoes, sweet potato and French shallots in a single layer in a large roasting tin. Place in the oven 20 minutes after the chicken and roast for 25 minutes, then add the zucchini, cut side down, and the garlic cloves. Cook for a further 25 minutes, or until golden and tender, turning the vegetables occasionally to ensure they don't burn. Discard the lemon and serve the chicken with the roast vegetables and peeled garlic cloves.

nutrition per serve: Energy 2483 kJ (593 Cal); Fat 27 g; Saturated fat 7.5 g; Protein 42.9 g; Carbohydrate 39.9 g; Fibre 8.4 g; Cholesterol 178 mg

BEEF AND HOKKIEN NOODLE STIR-FRY

600 g (1 lb 5 oz) fresh hokkien (egg) noodles
olive oil spray
350 g (12 oz) lean beef fillet, partially frozen, thinly sliced
1 tbsp peanut oil
1 large onion, cut into thin wedges
1 large carrot, thinly sliced on the diagonal
1 red capsicum (pepper), cut into thin strips
2 garlic cloves, crushed
1 tsp grated fresh ginger

100 g (3½ oz) snow peas (mangetout), sliced in half on the diagonal
200 g (7 oz) shiitake mushrooms, sliced
3 tbsp oyster sauce
2 tbsp light soy sauce
1 tbsp soft brown sugar
½ tsp five-spice powder

PREP TIME: 15 MINUTES
COOKING TIME: 15 MINUTES
SERVES 4

Put the noodles in a heatproof bowl with enough boiling water to cover. Leave to soften for 1 minute, separate the noodles with a fork, then drain and set aside.

Spray a large wok with oil and heat over high heat. Add the beef in batches and cook until brown. Remove and keep warm.

Heat the peanut oil in the wok, and when very hot, add the onion, carrot and capsicum and stir-fry for 2–3 minutes, or until tender. Add the garlic, ginger, snow peas and shiitake mushrooms and cook for another minute, then return the beef to the wok.

Add the noodles to the wok, tossing well. Combine the oyster sauce with the soy sauce, sugar, five-spice powder and 1 tablespoon water and pour over the noodles. Toss until warmed through and serve immediately.

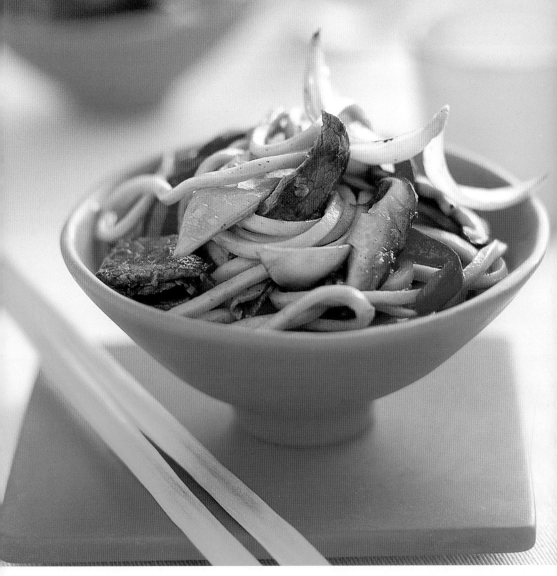

THE WHOLE FAMILY WILL ENJOY
THIS STIR-FRY, WHICH INCLUDES
A VARIETY OF COLOURFUL
VEGETABLES. HOKKIEN NOODLES
ARE THICK, FRESH NOODLES MADE
FROM EGG AND WHEAT. THEY
HAVE BEEN COOKED AND LIGHTLY
OILED BEFORE PACKAGING.

nutrition per serve: Energy 1727 kJ (413 Cal)
Fat 11 g
Saturated fat 3.1 g
Protein 27.7 g
Carbohydrate 47.6 g
Fibre 6.8 g
Cholesterol 59 mg

SEARED TUNA WITH SESAME GREENS

THE TUNA IN THIS RECIPE IS MARINATED AND SEARED SO THAT IT RETAINS ITS MOISTURE AND SOFT TEXTURE. THIS MEAL PROVIDES FILLING LEAN PROTEIN AND GOOD AMOUNTS OF HEALTHY OMEGA-3 FAT.

80 ml (2½ fl oz/⅓ cup) soy sauce
3 tbsp mirin
1 tbsp sake
1 tsp caster (superfine) sugar
1 tsp finely grated fresh ginger
2 tsp lemon juice
4 x 175 g (6 oz) tuna steaks
olive oil spray
350 g (12 oz/1 bunch) choy sum (Chinese flowering cabbage), trimmed and halved

800 g (1 lb 12 oz/1 bunch) Chinese broccoli (gai larn), trimmed and halved
2 tsp sesame seeds, lightly toasted

PREP TIME: 15 MINUTES + 30 MINUTES MARINATING
COOKING TIME: 10 MINUTES
SERVES 4

Combine the soy sauce, mirin, sake, sugar, ginger and lemon juice together in a bowl, stirring to dissolve the sugar. Put the tuna in a shallow non-metallic dish and spoon the soy marinade over the top. Turn the tuna in the marinade so it is well coated. Cover and leave to marinate in the refrigerator for 30 minutes.

Preheat a chargrill pan over high heat and spray with the oil. Lift the tuna out of the marinade, reserving the marinade. Cook the tuna for 1½–2 minutes on each side, until cooked on the outside but still pink in the middle.

Pour the marinade into a large frying pan. Bring the liquid to the boil, add the choy sum, Chinese broccoli and sesame seeds to the simmering sauce. Cook, turning the vegetables until lightly wilted, then place onto serving plates. Top the vegetables with the tuna and spoon the marinade over the top. Serve with rice or noodles.

HINTS:
• Sake, mirin and sesame oil are available in supermarkets and Asian stores. You can use any Asian-style vegetable such as bok choy (pak choy) or broccolini.
• As a variation, use salmon instead of the tuna.

nutrition per serve: Energy 1598 kJ (382 Cal); Fat 11.8 g; Saturated fat 4.2 g; Protein 50.9 g; Carbohydrate 11.2 g; Fibre 8.2 g; Cholesterol 63 mg

THAI CHICKEN BURGERS

THESE ASIAN-STYLE BURGERS ARE DELICIOUSLY DIFFERENT FROM THE RUN-OF-THE MILL TYPE. CHANGING THE BREAD ROLLS FROM THE USUAL WHITE BREAD TO WHOLEGRAIN ADDS MORE FIBRE.

400 g (14 oz) lean minced (ground) chicken
80 g (2¾ oz/1 cup) fresh wholegrain
   breadcrumbs
1 garlic clove, crushed
1 large handful coriander (cilantro) leaves,
   chopped, plus 1 tbsp extra
3 tbsp sweet chilli sauce
1 tsp ground coriander
3 spring onions (scallions), finely chopped
60 g (2¼ oz/¼ cup) sugar
2 tbsp white vinegar
2 tbsp finely chopped raw or dry-roasted
   peanuts

1 large carrot
1 large Lebanese (short) cucumber
olive oil spray
4 wholegrain flat bread rolls or buns
2 handfuls mixed lettuce leaves
1 vine-ripened tomato, sliced

PREP TIME: 25 MINUTES + 30 MINUTES
   REFRIGERATION
COOKING TIME: 15 MINUTES
SERVES 4

Put the chicken, breadcrumbs, garlic, coriander, chilli sauce, ground coriander and spring onion in a large bowl. Mix together with your hands. Shape the mixture into four patties and then refrigerate, covered, for 30 minutes.

To make the dressing, put the sugar, vinegar and 3 tablespoons water in a small saucepan and stir over low heat until the sugar dissolves. Simmer for 5 minutes, or until slightly thickened. Cool and stir in the peanuts and extra coriander. Peel strips of carrot and cucumber to make 'ribbons' and set aside.

Heat a heavy-based frying pan or barbecue hotplate to high, spray with the oil and cook the chicken burgers for 4 minutes on each side, or until cooked through. Serve on toasted bread rolls or buns, with the dressing, carrot and cucumber ribbons, lettuce and tomato.

HINTS:
• To save time, make a batch of the chicken patties on the weekend and freeze them individually. Pull them out when you are ready to eat them. They will freeze for 1 month.
• Wholegrain hamburger buns may be difficult to find, so use wholegrain bread rolls or thick slices of wholegrain bread.

nutrition per serve: Energy 1957 kJ (468 Cal); Fat 12.2 g; Saturated fat 2.6 g; Protein 25.3 g; Carbohydrate 56.9 g; Fibre 14.4 g; Cholesterol 78 mg

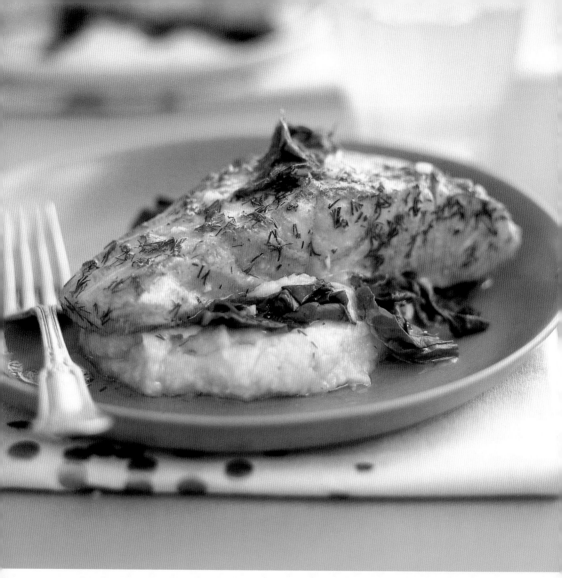

THIS IS AN EXCELLENT RECIPE
AS IT INCLUDES BOTH FISH AND
LEGUMES—TWO OF THE FOODS
MOST PEOPLE DON'T EAT
ENOUGH OF. IT ALSO PROVIDES
LEAN PROTEIN AND SLOWLY
DIGESTED CARBOHYDRATE.

nutrition per serve: Energy 1710 kJ (409 Cal)
Fat 15.9 g
Saturated fat 3.2 mg
Protein 47.1 g
Carbohydrate 15.1 g
Fibre 10.2 g
Cholesterol 95 mg

SALMON WITH BEAN PUREE

4 x 180 g (6 oz) salmon fillets
2 tsp canola oil
1 garlic clove, crushed
2 tbsp white wine vinegar
1 tsp finely grated lime zest
2 tbsp chopped dill
600 g (1 lb 5 oz) tinned cannellini beans,
   drained and rinsed, to yield about 380 g
   (13½ oz) drained beans

1 bay leaf
250 ml (9 fl oz/1 cup) chicken stock
500 g (1 lb 2 oz/1 bunch) baby English
   spinach leaves, roughly chopped

PREP TIME: 15 MINUTES + 10 MINUTES
   MARINATING
COOKING TIME: 25 MINUTES
SERVES 4

Put the salmon in a non-metallic dish. Combine the oil, garlic, vinegar, lime zest and dill, pour over the fish, then cover and leave to marinate for 10 minutes.

Put the beans, bay leaf and stock in a saucepan, bring to the boil, then reduce the heat and simmer for 10 minutes. Remove the bay leaf. Cool a little, then transfer to a food processor and purée. Season well with salt and freshly ground black pepper.

Drain the salmon, reserving the marinade. Heat a non-stick frying pan over high heat, add the salmon and cook for 3–5 minutes on each side, or until crisp and golden. Remove from the pan and set aside. Add the marinade to the pan and bring to the boil.

Steam the spinach until wilted. Place a mound of bean purée on each serving plate and top with the wilted spinach and salmon fillets. Drizzle over the marinade. Serve with chunky slices of brown bread and a side dish of steamed squash or sweet corn.

ROSEMARY LAMB WITH BEANS

This Mediterranean-style meal will satisfy the heartiest of appetites—it provides plenty of fibre, protein and low-GI starch, and is a good source of iron, zinc, niacin and folate.

2 tomatoes
375 g (13 oz) small shell pasta
600 g (1 lb 5 oz) lean lamb fillet
olive oil spray
3 garlic cloves, finely chopped
1 tsp cumin seeds
2 tsp finely chopped rosemary
2 tbsp red wine vinegar

1 tbsp lemon juice
300 g (10½ oz) tinned cannellini beans, drained and rinsed
2 tbsp chopped flat-leaf (Italian) parsley

Prep time: 20 minutes
Cooking time: 20 minutes
Serves 4

To peel the tomatoes, score a cross in the base of each tomato. Put in a heatproof bowl and cover with boiling water. Leave for 30 seconds, then transfer to cold water and peel the skin away from the cross. Cut into quarters, scoop out the seeds with a teaspoon and finely chop the flesh into cubes.

Cook the shell pasta in a large saucepan of boiling water for 10 minutes, or until *al dente*. Drain well.

Trim the lamb, then thinly slice it on the diagonal. Heat a large frying pan until very hot and spray with the oil. Add the lamb in two batches and cook over very high heat, stirring frequently until browned. Return all the lamb to the pan, then add the garlic, cumin and rosemary. Cook for 1 minute, then reduce the heat and pour in the vinegar and lemon juice. Stir to combine, scraping up any sediment from the bottom of the pan.

Add the tomato and cannellini beans and stir until warmed through. Season with salt and freshly ground black pepper, then scatter with the parsley. Serve with the pasta.

nutrition per serve: Energy 2370 kJ (566 Cal); Fat 7.8 g; Saturated fat 2.8 g; Protein 46.2 g; Carbohydrate 72.6 g; Fibre 8 g; Cholesterol 97 mg

BEEF STROGANOFF

THIS RECIPE CONTAINS LESS FAT THAN THE REGULAR VERSION, BUT IS STILL RICH IN FLAVOUR. USING EVAPORATED MILK INSTEAD OF CREAM CUTS LOTS OF FAT WHILE STILL PRODUCING A DELICIOUS CREAMY SAUCE.

500 g (1 lb 2 oz) lean beef rump steak
olive oil spray
1 onion, sliced
¼ tsp paprika
250 g (9 oz) button mushrooms, halved
2 tbsp tomato paste (concentrated purée)
125 ml (4 fl oz/½ cup) beef stock
375 g (13 oz) fettucine

125 ml (4 fl oz/½ cup) evaporated skim milk
3 tsp cornflour (cornstarch)
3 tbsp chopped parsley

PREP TIME: 20 MINUTES

COOKING TIME: 30 MINUTES

SERVES 4

Trim the beef and slice it into thin strips. Heat a large non-stick frying pan over high heat and spray with the oil. Add the beef in batches and cook for 2–3 minutes, or until just cooked. Remove from the pan.

Lightly spray the pan with oil again and cook the onion, paprika and mushrooms over medium heat until the onion has softened. Add the beef, tomato paste, stock and 125 ml (4 fl oz/½ cup) water. Bring to the boil, then reduce the heat and simmer for 10 minutes.

Meanwhile, cook the pasta in a large saucepan of boiling water for 10 minutes, or until *al dente*. Drain well.

Mix the evaporated milk with the cornflour in a small bowl. Add to the pan and stir until the sauce boils and thickens. Sprinkle with parsley and serve with the fettucine. Serve with a salad or steamed vegetables.

HINT:
• To increase the fibre content further, use wholemeal (whole-wheat) pasta.

nutrition per serve: Energy 2386 kJ (570 Cal); Fat 8.1 g; Saturated fat 2.9 g; Protein 45.3 g; Carbohydrate 75 g; Fibre 5 g; Cholesterol 99 mg

PORK, BOK CHOY AND BLACK BEAN STIR-FRY

300 g (10½ oz/1½ cups) brown basmati
  rice, rinsed and drained

400 g (14 oz) lean pork leg steaks

2 tsp sesame oil

2 onions, thinly sliced

2 garlic cloves, finely chopped

2–3 tsp chopped fresh ginger

1 red capsicum (pepper), cut into strips

1 tbsp salted black beans, rinsed, roughly
  chopped

500 g (1 lb 2 oz) baby bok choy (pak choy),
  shredded

80 g (2¾ oz/½ cup) drained and rinsed
  tinned water chestnuts, thinly sliced

2 tbsp oyster sauce

1 tbsp soy sauce

2 tsp fish sauce

PREP TIME: 20 MINUTES

COOKING TIME: 1 HOUR

SERVES 4

Put 1.5 litres (52 fl oz/6 cups) water in a saucepan and bring to the boil over medium heat. Add the rice and cook for 30–35 minutes, stirring occasionally, until the rice is tender.

Meanwhile, slice the pork into strips across the grain. Heat a wok over medium–high heat, add half the sesame oil and swirl to coat the wok. Add the onion, garlic and ginger to the wok and cook for 3–4 minutes, being careful that the garlic doesn't burn. Add the capsicum and cook for 2–3 minutes. Remove from the wok.

Heat the remaining sesame oil in the wok, add the pork in batches and briefly stir-fry until browned. Reheat the wok between batches.

Return all the pork to the wok along with the capsicum mixture, black beans, bok choy and water chestnuts. Stir in the oyster sauce, soy sauce and fish sauce. Toss quickly, reduce the heat, then cover and steam for 3–4 minutes, or until the bok choy has just wilted. Serve the stir-fry with the brown rice.

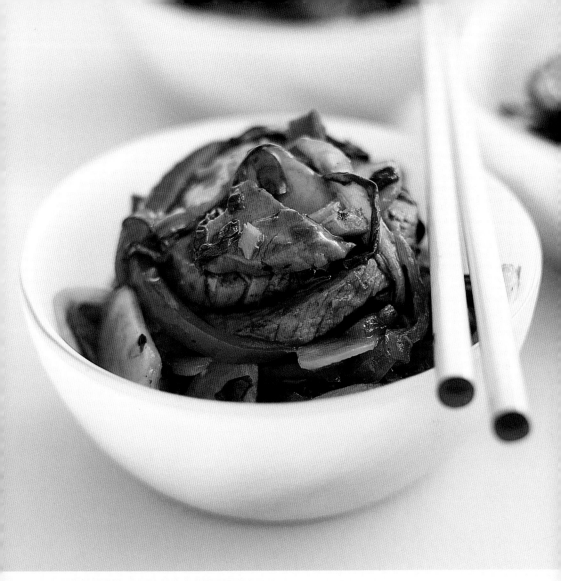

BY MAKING SIMPLE CHANGES, SUCH AS SWAPPING WHITE RICE FOR BROWN, YOU CAN EASILY SLIP MORE FIBRE INTO YOUR DAILY MEALS, WITHOUT TOO MUCH EFFORT AT ALL.

nutrition per serve: Energy 2077 kJ (496 Cal)
Fat 8.3 g
Saturated fat 2 g
Protein 37.9 g
Carbohydrate 69.1 g
Fibre 6.3 g
Cholesterol 57 mg

SPAGHETTI WITH MEATBALLS

THIS CLASSIC RECIPE IS A FAMILY FAVOURITE. IT ALREADY PROVIDES GOOD AMOUNTS OF FIBRE FROM THE TOMATOES, PASTA AND BREADCRUMBS, BUT YOU CAN INCREASE THE FIBRE EVEN MORE BY USING WHOLEMEAL SPAGHETTI.

500 g (1 lb 2 oz) lean minced (ground) beef
40 g (1½ oz/½ cup) fresh wholegrain breadcrumbs
1 small onion, finely chopped
2 garlic cloves, crushed
2 tsp worcestershire sauce
1 tsp dried oregano
30 g (1 oz/¼ cup) plain (all-purpose) flour
1 tbsp olive oil
400 g (14 oz) spaghetti

SAUCE
2 x 400 g (14 oz) tins chopped tomatoes
1 tsp olive oil
1 onion, finely chopped
2 garlic cloves, crushed
2 tbsp tomato paste (concentrated purée)
125 ml (4 fl oz/½ cup) beef stock

PREP TIME: 30 MINUTES
COOKING TIME: 40 MINUTES
SERVES 4

To make the meatballs, combine the beef, breadcrumbs, onion, garlic, worcestershire sauce and oregano in a bowl. Season with salt and freshly ground black pepper. Use your hands to mix the ingredients together. Roll level tablespoons of the mixture into balls, dust lightly with the flour and shake off the excess.

Heat the oil in a deep frying pan and cook the meatballs in batches, turning frequently, until browned all over. Drain well on paper towels. Wipe the pan out with paper towels.

To make the sauce, purée the tomatoes in a food processor or blender. Heat the oil in the frying pan, add the onion and cook over medium heat for 2–3 minutes, or until soft and lightly golden. Add the garlic and cook for a further 1 minute. Add the puréed tomatoes, tomato paste and stock to the pan and stir to combine. Bring the mixture to the boil, then add the meatballs. Reduce the heat and simmer for 15 minutes, turning the meatballs once. Season with freshly ground black pepper.

Meanwhile, cook the spaghetti in a large saucepan of boiling water for 10 minutes, or until *al dente*. Drain well, then divide among four plates and top with the meatballs and sauce. Serve with a mixed green salad.

nutrition per serve: Energy 2899 kJ (693 Cal); Fat 16.4 g; Saturated fat 4.7 g; Protein 41.6 g; Carbohydrate 89.1 g; Fibre 8.2 g; Cholesterol 64 mg

BEEF AND VEGETABLE CURRY

THIS SLOW-COOKED AROMATIC CURRY IS A GREAT MEAL FOR WEEKENDS, WHEN YOU'VE GOT TIME. THIS DISH PROVIDES IRON, ZINC AND B-GROUP VITAMINS AND IS RICH IN BETA-CAROTENE AND FOLATE.

2 tsp olive oil
1 large onion, chopped
2 garlic cloves, crushed
1 tbsp grated fresh ginger
2 tsp chopped red chilli
2 tsp ground cumin
2 tsp ground coriander
1 tsp ground cardamom
1 tsp ground turmeric
1/2 tsp ground cloves
750 g (1 lb 10 oz) lean beef, such as chuck
   or blade, cubed

400 g (14 oz) tin crushed tomatoes
250 ml (9 fl oz/1 cup) beef stock
650 g (1 lb 7 oz) unpeeled potatoes, cut
   into large chunks
125 g (4 1/2 oz) green beans, sliced
2 carrots, sliced
125 g (4 1/2 oz/1/2 cup) low-fat plain yoghurt

PREP TIME: 30 MINUTES
COOKING TIME: 2 1/2 HOURS
SERVES 4

Heat the oil in a large pan, add the onion and cook over low heat for 15 minutes, stirring regularly, until soft. Add the garlic, ginger, chilli and spices and stir for 1 minute.

Add the beef and stir to coat with the spices. Add the tomatoes and beef stock and bring to the boil. Reduce the heat to very low, cover and simmer for 1 1/2 hours.

Add the potato and cook for a further 25 minutes, then uncover, add the beans and carrots and cook for 15 minutes, or until the vegetables are tender and the sauce thickens. Stir in the yoghurt, heat through and serve with white or brown basmati rice.

nutrition per serve: Energy 1941 kJ (464 Cal); Fat 12 g; Saturated fat 4.2 g; Protein 49.4 g; Carbohydrate 34.3 g; Fibre 8.2 g; Cholesterol 112 mg

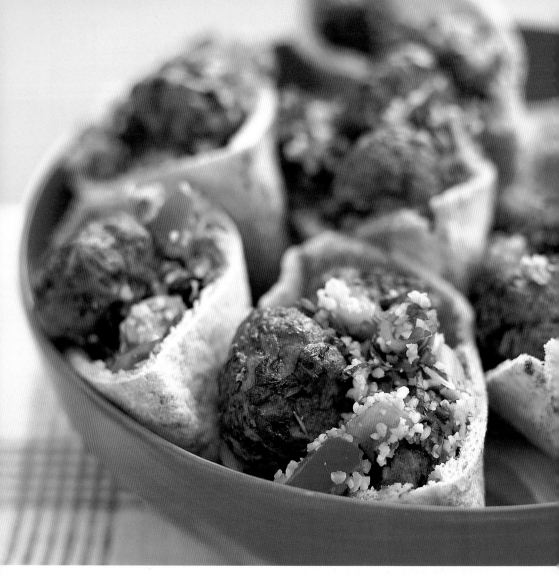

THIS MEAL IS AN EASY ONE TO
PREPARE AND IS LOWER IN FAT
AND KILOJOULES THAN THE
TAKEAWAY VERSION. THIS IS A
GREAT HIGH-FIBRE RECIPE THAT
CHILDREN WILL ALSO ENJOY.

nutrition per serve: Energy 2200 kJ (525 Cal)

Fat 8.1 g

Saturated fat 2.6 g

Protein 40.5 g

Carbohydrate 63.9 g

Fibre 12 g

Cholesterol 84 mg

LAMB KOFTAS IN PITTA BREAD

500 g (1 lb 2 oz) lean lamb
1 onion, roughly chopped
1 large handful flat-leaf (Italian)
  parsley, roughly chopped
1 large handful mint, roughly
  chopped
2 tsp lemon zest
1 tsp ground cumin
¼ tsp chilli powder
250 g (9 oz/1 cup) low-fat plain
  yoghurt
2 tsp lemon juice
olive oil spray
4 wholemeal (whole-wheat)
  pitta breads

TABOULEH
90 g (3¼ oz/½ cup) burghul (bulgur)
2 vine-ripened tomatoes
1 Lebanese (short) cucumber
60 g (2¼ oz/½ bunch) flat-leaf
  (Italian) parsley, chopped
1 large handful mint, chopped
2 French shallots, chopped
125 ml (4 fl oz/½ cup) fat-free Greek
  or Italian dressing

PREP TIME: 35 MINUTES + 30 MINUTES
  RESTING
COOKING TIME: 15 MINUTES
SERVES 4

Roughly chop the lamb. Put the lamb and onion in a food processor and process until smooth. Add the parsley, mint, lemon zest and spices and process until well combined. Divide the mixture into 24 balls and place on a tray. Cover and refrigerate for at least 30 minutes for the flavours to develop.

Meanwhile, to make the tabouleh, put the burghul in a bowl. Cover with boiling water, set aside for 10 minutes, or until softened. Drain, then use clean hands to squeeze dry. Cut the tomatoes in half, scoop out the seeds with a teaspoon, then chop the flesh. Cut the cucumber in halves lengthways, scoop out the seeds, then chop the flesh. Put the burghul, tomato and cucumber in a large bowl with the parsley, mint and shallots. Stir in the dressing.

To make the yoghurt dressing, combine the yoghurt and lemon juice in a bowl. Cover and refrigerate until needed.

Heat a large, non-stick frying pan over medium heat and spray with the oil. Cook the lamb balls in two batches, spraying the pan with oil before each batch, until browned all over and cooked through.

Preheat the oven to 180°C (350°F/Gas 4). Cut the pitta breads in half, wrap in foil and place in the oven for 10 minutes to warm. To serve, divide the tabouleh among the pitta bread halves, add three kofta balls to each and top with the yoghurt dressing.

SPAGHETTI MARINARA

IT'S IMPORTANT TO INCLUDE SEAFOOD IN OUR DIET AND THIS RECIPE MAKES THAT EASY. IF YOU ARE SHORT ON TIME, SUBSTITUTE 500 G (1 LB 2 OZ) FRESH OR FROZEN MARINARA MIX FOR THE MUSSELS, SQUID, FISH AND PRAWNS.

125 g (4½ oz) small squid hoods
125 g (4½ oz) skinless firm white
   fish fillets
200 g (7 oz) raw prawns (shrimp)
12 mussels
2 tsp olive oil
1 onion, chopped
2 garlic cloves, crushed
125 ml (4 fl oz/½ cup) red wine
2 tbsp tomato paste (concentrated purée)
400 g (14 oz) tin chopped tomatoes

250 ml (9 fl oz/1 cup) bottled tomato
   pasta sauce
1 tbsp chopped basil
1 tbsp chopped oregano
20 g (¾ oz) canola margarine
500 g (1 lb 2 oz) spaghetti

PREP TIME: 50 MINUTES
COOKING TIME: 30 MINUTES
SERVES 4

To prepare the seafood, slice the squid hoods into rings. Cut the fish into bite-sized cubes, checking for bones. Peel the prawns, leaving the tails intact. Gently pull out the dark vein from each prawn back, starting at the head end. Scrub the mussels with a stiff brush and pull out the hairy beards. Discard any mussels that are broken or any open ones that don't close when tapped on the bench.

Heat the olive oil in a large saucepan. Add the onion and garlic and cook over low heat for 2–3 minutes. Increase the heat to medium and add the wine, tomato paste, tomatoes and pasta sauce. Simmer, stirring occasionally, for 5–10 minutes, or until the sauce reduces and thickens slightly. Stir in the herbs and season to taste. Keep warm.

While the sauce is simmering, heat 125 ml (4 fl oz/½ cup) water in a saucepan. Add the mussels, cover and steam for 3–5 minutes, or until the mussels have opened. Remove the mussels from the pan, discarding any that haven't opened, and stir the liquid left in the pan into the tomato sauce.

Heat the margarine in a frying pan and sauté the squid, fish and prawns in batches for 1–2 minutes, or until cooked. Add the seafood to the warm tomato sauce and stir gently.

Meanwhile, cook the pasta in a large saucepan of boiling water for 10 minutes, or until al dente. Drain and toss with the seafood sauce. Serve immediately with a green salad.

nutrition per serve: Energy 2790 kJ (664 Cal); Fat 10 g; Saturated fat 3.9 g; Protein 39.5 g; Carbohydrate 97.5 g; Fibre 7.9 g; Cholesterol 154 mg

PEPPERED LAMB, ASPARAGUS AND BROCCOLI STIR-FRY

THE BROWN RICE TOGETHER WITH THE BEEF AND VEGETABLES MAKES A VERY FILLING MEAL. BASMATI IS A LONG-GRAIN RICE, AVAILABLE BOTH AS A WHITE AND BROWN RICE.

2 tsp green peppercorns, finely chopped
3 garlic cloves, finely chopped
1 tbsp canola oil
400 g (14 oz) lean lamb fillets, trimmed
300 g (10½ oz/1½ cups) brown basmati rice, rinsed and drained
canola oil spray
1 onion, cut into small wedges
80 ml (2½ fl oz/⅓ cup) dry sherry
1 green capsicum (pepper), cut into strips
20 small asparagus spears, trimmed and cut into bite-sized pieces
250 g (9 oz) broccoli florets
50 g (1¾ oz/⅓ cup) tinned or frozen soya beans
2 tbsp oyster sauce
garlic chives, snipped into short lengths, to garnish

PREP TIME: 20 MINUTES + 20 MINUTES MARINATING
COOKING TIME: 55 MINUTES
SERVES 4

To make the marinade, put the green peppercorns, garlic and oil in a large bowl. Add the trimmed lamb and toss well to coat. Cover with plastic wrap and marinate for 20 minutes.

Put 1.5 litres (52 fl oz/6 cups) water in a saucepan and bring to the boil over medium heat. Add the rice and cook for 30–35 minutes, stirring occasionally, until the rice is tender.

Remove the lamb from the marinade and cut into bite-sized pieces. Spray a wok with oil and heat over high heat until slightly smoking. Add the lamb in small batches and stir-fry briefly until browned and just cooked. Remove from the wok and keep warm. Reheat the wok between batches.

Reheat the wok, spray with oil and stir-fry the onion and 2 teaspoons of the sherry for 1 minute. Add the capsicum and a large pinch of salt. Cover, steam for 2 minutes, then add the asparagus, broccoli and the remaining sherry and stir-fry for 1 minute. Cover and steam for 3 minutes, or until the vegetables are just tender. Return the lamb to the wok along with the soya beans to heat through, add the oyster sauce and stir to combine with the vegetables. Garnish with the chives and serve with the brown rice.

nutrition per serve: Energy 2241 kJ (535 Cal); Fat 11.8 g; Saturated fat 2.5 g; Protein 33.1 g; Carbohydrate 64.9 g; Fibre 7.5 g; Cholesterol 65 mg

STEAK SANDWICH WITH ONION RELISH

RED ONION RELISH
1 tsp olive oil
2 red onions, thinly sliced
2 tbsp soft brown sugar
2 tbsp balsamic vinegar
1 tbsp thyme

2 tsp olive oil
250 g (9 oz) mixed mushrooms
(flat, button, shiitake), sliced

olive oil spray
4 x 60 g (2¼ oz) lean minute beef steaks, trimmed
125 g (4½ oz) baby English spinach leaves
8 slices wholegrain bread
1 large tomato, sliced

PREP TIME: 20 MINUTES
COOKING TIME: 25 MINUTES
SERVES 4

To make the red onion relish, heat the oil in a saucepan, add the onion and cook over low heat for 10 minutes, or until softened, stirring frequently and taking care not to burn. Add the sugar and balsamic vinegar and cook, stirring, for 10–12 minutes, or until softened and slightly syrupy. Stir in the thyme.

Meanwhile, heat the olive oil in a heavy-based frying pan over medium heat. Stir in the mushrooms, then add 2 tablespoons water. Cover, then reduce the heat and simmer for 5 minutes, or until softened, making sure the mushrooms don't dry out. Stir once or twice. Remove the lid and increase the heat to allow any juice to evaporate. Season well with freshly ground black pepper.

Lightly spray a chargrill pan or frying pan with the oil. Add the steak and cook for 1 minute on each side, or until cooked to your liking. Very briefly microwave or steam the spinach until just wilted. Drain away any juices.

Toast the bread and arrange one slice of toast on each plate. Top with the spinach, then the steak, mushrooms and tomato and finish with a dollop of the onion relish. Top with the remaining slice of toast. Serve with a mixed green salad.

HINT:
• For full flavour, use at least two varieties of mushrooms.

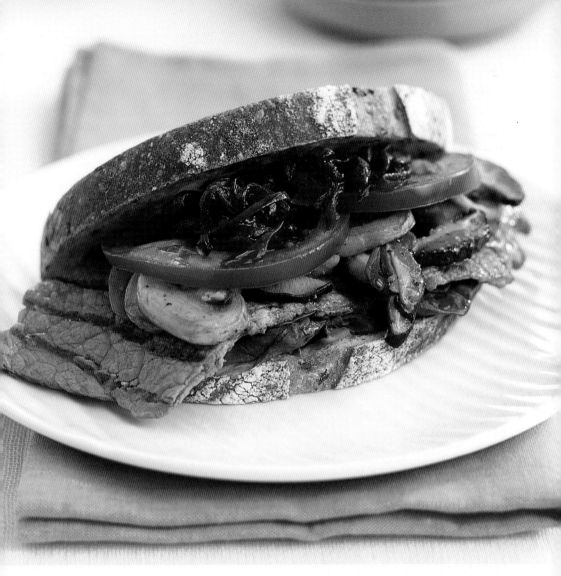

IT'S EASY TO JAZZ UP A SIMPLE
STEAK SANDWICH TO MAKE IT
MORE NUTRITIOUS AND
DELICIOUS—SIMPLY USE GRAINY
BREAD AND LEAN MEAT AND ADD
A TASTY HOME-MADE RELISH AND
SOME VEGETABLES.

nutrition per serve: Energy 1454 kJ (347 Cal)
Fat 8.7 g
Saturated fat 1.8 g
Protein 23.1 g
Carbohydrate 40 g
Fibre 7.6 g
Cholesterol 34 mg

131

SHEPHERD'S PIE

This pie is a great family meal and is an excellent choice for children, providing good amounts of carbohydrate, protein, b-group vitamins, fibre, iron and zinc.

olive oil spray

2 onions, thinly sliced

1 large carrot, finely chopped

2 celery stalks, finely chopped

500 g (1 lb 2 oz) lean minced (ground) lamb

2 tbsp plain (all-purpose) flour

2 tbsp tomato paste (concentrated purée)

2 tbsp worcestershire sauce

1 beef or chicken stock cube

1.25 kg (2 lb 12 oz) potatoes, peeled and chopped

125 ml (4 fl oz/½ cup) skim milk

2 large handfuls parsley, finely chopped

paprika, to sprinkle

Prep time: 20 minutes

Cooking time: 50 minutes

Serves 4

Lightly spray a large non-stick frying pan with oil and heat over medium heat. Add the onion, carrot and celery and cook, stirring constantly, for 5 minutes, or until the vegetables begin to soften. Add 1 tablespoon water to prevent sticking. Remove from the pan and set aside. Spray the pan with a little more oil, add the lamb and cook, stirring, over high heat until well browned.

Add the flour and stir for 2–3 minutes. Return the vegetables to the pan along with the tomato paste, worcestershire sauce, stock cube and 500 ml (17 fl oz/2 cups) water. Slowly bring to the boil. Reduce the heat, cover and simmer for 20 minutes, stirring occasionally.

Meanwhile, steam or microwave the potato until tender. Drain and mash until smooth. Add the milk, season with salt and freshly ground black pepper and beat well.

Stir the parsley through the lamb and season. Preheat a grill (broiler). Pour the lamb into a 1.5 litre (52 fl oz/6 cup) heatproof dish. Spoon the mashed potato over the top and spread it evenly with the back of the spoon. Use a fork to roughen up the potato. Sprinkle with paprika and grill (broil) until the potato is golden, watching carefully because the potato browns quickly. Serve with a green salad.

nutrition per serve: Energy 1874 kJ (448 Cal); Fat 9.8 g; Saturated fat 3.8 g; Protein 35.4 g; Carbohydrate 49.7 g; Fibre 7 g; Cholesterol 65 mg

RIGATONI WITH KIDNEY BEANS AND SAUSAGE

THIS RECIPE COMBINES LEGUMES AND SAUSAGES FOR A TASTY AND FILLING LOW-GI MEAL. CHOOSE GOOD-QUALITY LEAN SAUSAGES TO KEEP THE FAT CONTENT LOW.

2 tsp olive oil
1 large onion, chopped
2 garlic cloves, crushed
4 lean beef sausages
2 x 400 g (14 oz) tins chopped tomatoes
400 g (14 oz) tin red kidney beans, drained
    and rinsed
2 tbsp chopped basil
1 tbsp chopped sage

1 tbsp chopped parsley
500 g (1 lb 2 oz) rigatoni
grated parmesan cheese, to serve
    (optional)

PREP TIME: 25 MINUTES
COOKING TIME: 35 MINUTES
SERVES 4–6

Heat the oil in a large saucepan over medium heat. Add the onion, garlic and sausages and cook, stirring occasionally, for 5 minutes. Remove the sausages, chop them and return to the saucepan.

Add the tomatoes, kidney beans, basil, sage and parsley and season well with salt and freshly ground black pepper. Reduce the heat and simmer for 20 minutes.

Meanwhile, cook the pasta in a large saucepan of boiling water for 10 minutes, or until *al dente*. Drain well. Divide among bowls and top with the sauce. If you like, sprinkle with parmesan before serving.

HINTS:
• If you prefer, you can use dried kidney beans instead of the tinned ones. Soak them overnight in water, then drain, transfer to a saucepan, cover well with water and boil for 20 minutes, or until tender.
• Any large pasta shape will work well. Use wholemeal (whole-wheat) pasta instead of white to raise the fibre content even more.
• Any leftovers can be frozen or stored in the refrigerator for up to 3 days.

nutrition per serve (6): Energy 1866 kJ (446 Cal); Fat 6.7 g; Saturated fat 1.7 g; Protein 19.8 g; Carbohydrate 72.8 g; Fibre 7.7 g; Cholesterol 23 mg

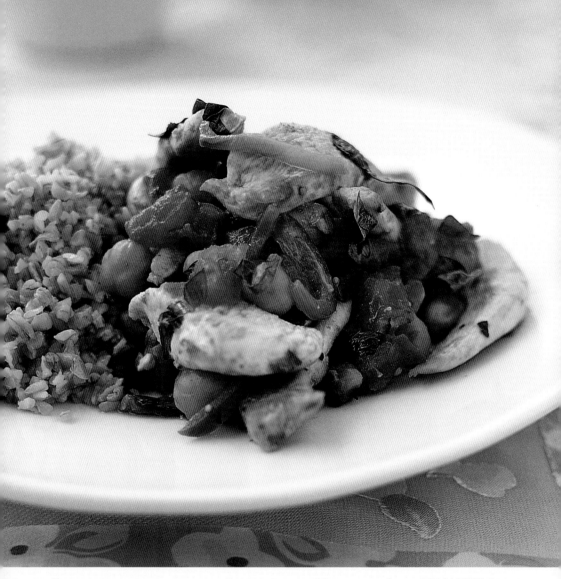

THIS IS A NOURISHING MEAL
THAT TASTES GREAT AND IS
EASY TO MAKE. BURGHUL AND
CHICKPEAS ARE BOTH LOW GI
AND ARE EXCELLENT SOURCES
OF INSOLUBLE FIBRE.

nutrition per serve: Energy 2456 kJ (587 Cal)

Fat 13.7 g

Saturated fat 2.2 g

Protein 39.5 g

Carbohydrate 63.3 g

Fibre 20.7 g

Cholesterol 65 mg

MIDDLE-EASTERN CHICKEN WITH BURGHUL

350 g (12 oz/2 cups) burghul (bulgur)
2 boneless skinless chicken breasts
2 tsp olive oil
1 red onion, thinly sliced
300 g (10½ oz) tin chickpeas, drained and rinsed
70 g (2½ oz/½ cup) unsalted pistachio kernels
1 tomato, chopped

juice of 1 orange
4 tbsp finely chopped flat-leaf (Italian) parsley

PREP TIME: 15 MINUTES + 15 MINUTES SOAKING

COOKING TIME: 20 MINUTES

SERVES 4

Put the burghul in a bowl, cover with water and leave to soak for 15 minutes, or until the burghul has softened. Drain and use clean hands to squeeze dry.

Meanwhile, trim the chicken and thinly slice. Heat a large frying pan over high heat, add half the oil and swirl to coat. Add the chicken in batches and stir-fry for 3–5 minutes, or until cooked. Remove from the pan and keep warm. Reheat the pan between batches.

Add the remaining oil to the pan and cook the onion, stirring, for 2 minutes, then add the chickpeas, pistachios and tomato. Cook, stirring, for 3–5 minutes, or until the chickpeas are warmed through.

Pour in the orange juice, return the chicken and its juices to the pan and cook until half the juice has evaporated. Stir in the parsley. Season well with salt and freshly ground black pepper and serve with the burghul.

VEGETARIAN
MEALS

SOBA NOODLES WITH TOFU AND MUSHROOMS

SOBA NOODLES ARE MADE FROM BUCKWHEAT, A NUTTY-FLAVOURED GRAIN, AND SOME MAY CONTAIN ADDED WHEAT FLOUR. THE MARINATED TOFU TEAMS WELL WITH THE VARIED TEXTURES OF THE NOODLES AND VEGETABLES.

2 tsp sesame oil

3 tbsp light soy sauce

2 tbsp mirin

2 garlic cloves, finely chopped

2 tsp finely chopped fresh ginger

300 g (10½ oz) packet firm tofu, drained and cut into 3 cm (1¼ in) cubes

300 g (10½ oz/½ bunch) Chinese broccoli (gai larn)

280 g (10 oz) packet soba (buckwheat) noodles

115 g (4 oz) fresh baby corn, trimmed

1 tsp canola oil

4 red Asian shallots, chopped

150 g (5½ oz) field mushrooms, thickly sliced

2 tsp sesame seeds, lightly toasted

PREP TIME: 15 MINUTES + 15 MINUTES MARINATING

COOKING TIME: 15 MINUTES

SERVES 4

Combine the sesame oil, soy sauce, mirin, garlic and ginger in a large non-metallic bowl. Add the tofu and gently coat in the marinade. Set aside for at least 15 minutes.

Trim the Chinese broccoli, wash and drain, then cut into 5 cm (2 in) pieces. Set aside.

Put the soba noodles in a large saucepan of cold water and bring to the boil. Add 250 ml (9 fl oz/1 cup) cold water, bring to the boil again and cook for 5 minutes. Drain. Blanch the corn in a saucepan of boiling water for 2 minutes, refresh in cold water and drain.

Heat the oil in a large non-stick wok. Add the shallots and mushrooms and stir-fry for 2–3 minutes. Add the Chinese broccoli and corn to the wok with 80 ml (2½ fl oz/⅓ cup) water. Stir-fry for a further 2 minutes, or until the Chinese broccoli is just wilted. Add the tofu and marinade and gently stir-fry until combined and heated through. Scatter with sesame seeds and serve on a bed of soba noodles.

HINTS:
• You can use any Asian green vegetable, such as baby bok choy (pak choy) or choy sum (Chinese flowering cabbage) instead of the Chinese broccoli.
• Mirin is available from supermarkets and Asian stores. Use dry sherry if unavailable.

nutrition per serve: Energy 1874 kJ (448 Cal); Fat 10.4 g; Saturated fat 1.4 g; Protein 24.5 g; Carbohydrate 61.8 g; Fibre 9.3 g; Cholesterol 0 mg

SPICED LENTIL AND RICE PILAFF

THIS WHOLESOME AROMATIC DISH PROVIDES FIBRE, ANTIOXIDANTS, IRON AND
ESSENTIAL AMINO ACIDS. SERVE AS A SIDE DISH OR AS A MEAL BY ITSELF.

**200 g (7 oz/1 cup) puy lentils or tiny
blue-green lentils**
2 tsp olive oil
1 small red chilli, seeded and chopped
2 garlic cloves, chopped
2 tsp grated fresh ginger
1 red onion, chopped
**1 small red capsicum (pepper),
chopped**
1 tsp garam masala

1 tsp ground turmeric
150 g (5½ oz/¾ cup) brown basmati rice
**1 litre (35 fl oz/4 cups) hot vegetable stock
or water**
155 g (5½ oz/1 cup) frozen peas, thawed

PREP TIME: 10 MINUTES + 1 HOUR SOAKING
COOKING TIME: 45 MINUTES
SERVES 4

Put the lentils in a bowl, cover with water and soak for 1 hour. Drain.

Heat the oil in a deep heavy-based frying pan. Add the chilli, garlic and ginger and cook
for 1 minute, then add the onion and capsicum. Cook, stirring, for 2–3 minutes, or until
softened. Add the garam masala and turmeric and cook, stirring, for 1 minute.

Stir in the lentils, rice and hot stock or water. Continue stirring and bring to the boil, then
reduce the heat, cover and simmer for 40 minutes, or until the lentils and rice are cooked.
Stir in the peas and heat through. Serve with a mixed salad.

HINT:
• Puy lentils are available at most delicatessens and some large supermarkets. They work
well in this dish because they hold their shape when cooked and won't break down to a
mash, even if overcooked.

nutrition per serve: Energy 1534 kJ (366 Cal); Fat 4.9 g; Saturated fat 0.8 g; Protein 18.5 g;
Carbohydrate 57.4 g; Fibre 11.6 g; Cholesterol 0 mg

TAGLIATELLE WITH ASPARAGUS, PEAS AND HERB SAUCE

375 g (13 oz) dried or 500 g (1 lb 2 oz) fresh
    tagliatelle
250 ml (9 fl oz/1 cup) vegetable stock
2 leeks, white part only, thinly sliced
3 garlic cloves, crushed
235 g (8½ oz/1½ cups) shelled fresh peas
1 tbsp finely chopped mint
400 g (14 oz) asparagus spears, ends
    trimmed, cut into 5 cm (2 in) lengths
1 large handful flat-leaf (Italian) parsley,
    finely chopped

2 handfuls basil, shredded
80 ml (2½ fl oz/⅓ cup) light cream
pinch of ground nutmeg
1 tbsp grated parmesan cheese
1 tbsp extra virgin olive oil
extra grated parmesan, to garnish
    (optional)

PREP TIME: 20 MINUTES
COOKING TIME: 25 MINUTES
SERVES 4

Bring a large saucepan of salted water to the boil and cook the tagliatelle until *al dente*. Drain well.

Put 125 ml (4 fl oz/½ cup) of the stock and the leek in a large, deep frying pan. Cook over low heat, stirring often, for 4–5 minutes. Stir in the garlic, peas and mint and cook for 1 minute. Add the remaining stock and 125 ml (4 fl oz/½ cup) water and bring to the boil, then reduce the heat and simmer for 5 minutes.

Add the asparagus, parsley and basil and season well with salt and freshly ground black pepper. Simmer for a further 3–4 minutes, or until the asparagus is just tender. Gradually increase the heat to reduce the sauce to a light coating consistency. Stir in the cream, nutmeg and parmesan and adjust the seasoning, to taste.

Add the tagliatelle to the sauce and toss lightly to coat. Divide among individual serving bowls and drizzle with the extra virgin olive oil. Garnish with extra grated parmesan, if desired.

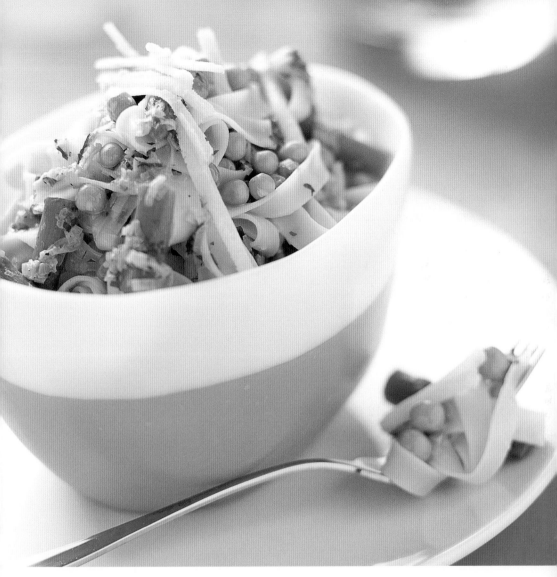

CELEBRATE THE RETURN OF SPRING
WITH THIS DISH USING FRESH,
IN-SEASON PEAS AND ASPARAGUS.
THIS LOW-GI, LOW-FAT DISH IS AN
EXCELLENT SOURCE OF FOLATE.

nutrition per serve: Energy 2093 kJ (500 Cal)
Fat 11.3 g
Saturated fat 4.2 g
Protein 19.5 g
Carbohydrate 74.6 g
Fibre 9.7 g
Cholesterol 15 mg

RATATOUILLE

RATATOUILLE IS NUTRITIOUS AND VERY VERSATILE. IT CAN BE SERVED HOT, COLD OR AT ROOM TEMPERATURE, AS A SIDE DISH OR AS A LIGHT MEAL WITH WHOLEGRAIN BREAD AND SALAD.

250 g (9 oz) eggplant (aubergine)
2 tbsp olive oil
250 g (9 oz) zucchini (courgettes), thickly
  sliced
2 onions, cut into wedges
1 red capsicum (pepper), cut into
  bite-sized cubes
1 green capsicum (pepper), cut into
  bite-sized cubes

2 garlic cloves, crushed
500 g (1 lb 2 oz) ripe tomatoes, chopped
1 tbsp chopped parsley
4 wholegrain bread rolls, to serve

PREP TIME: 20 MINUTES + 15 MINUTES
  STANDING
COOKING TIME: 40 MINUTES
SERVES 4

Thickly slice the eggplant, then spread it in a colander and sprinkle liberally with salt. Leave for 15 minutes, then rinse, pat dry with paper towels and cut into cubes.

Heat 1½ tablespoons of the oil in a large frying pan. Add the eggplant and zucchini in batches and cook for a few minutes, or until lightly browned. Drain well on paper towels.

Add the remaining oil to the pan and cook the onion over low heat for 3 minutes, or until golden. Add the red and green capsicums and cook for 5 minutes, or until tender but not browned. Add the garlic and tomatoes and cook, stirring, for 5 minutes.

Stir in the eggplant and zucchini. Simmer for 15–20 minutes to reduce and thicken the sauce. Stir in the parsley, then season to taste with salt and freshly ground black pepper. Serve with the wholegrain bread rolls.

HINT:
• Ratatouille is also delicious served as an accompaniment to rice or legumes, or with a chicken casserole and rice.

nutrition per serve: Energy 1545 kJ (369 Cal); Fat 12.9 g; Saturated fat 1.7 g; Protein 11.5 g; Carbohydrate 46.7 g; Fibre 9.9 g; Cholesterol <1 mg

LENTIL AND VEGETABLE CURRY

IF YOU LIKE A LITTLE SPICE IN YOUR MEALS, THIS DISH IS PERFECT. FOR EXTRA HEALTHY FIBRE, YOU CAN LEAVE THE VEGETABLES UNPEELED IF YOU LIKE—JUST GIVE THEM A GOOD WASH BEFORE COOKING.

1 tsp canola oil

1 large onion, chopped

2 garlic cloves, chopped

1–2 tbsp curry paste

1 tsp ground turmeric

200 g (7 oz/1 cup) green lentils, rinsed and drained

1.25 litres (44 fl oz/5 cups) vegetable stock or water

1 large carrot, peeled and cut into 2 cm (¾ in) cubes

2 potatoes, peeled and cut into 2 cm (¾ in) cubes

250 g (9 oz) sweet potato, peeled and cut into 2 cm (¾ in) cubes

350 g (12 oz) cauliflower, broken into small florets

150 g (5½ oz) green beans, trimmed and halved

basil, to serve

coriander (cilantro) leaves, to serve

PREP TIME: 20 MINUTES

COOKING TIME: 1 HOUR 10 MINUTES

SERVES 4

Heat the oil in a saucepan over medium heat. Add the onion and garlic and cook for 3 minutes, or until softened. Stir in the curry paste and turmeric and cook for 1 minute. Add the lentils and stock or water and bring to the boil. Reduce the heat, cover and simmer for 30 minutes, then add the carrot, potato and sweet potato. Simmer, covered, for a further 20 minutes, or until the lentils and vegetables are tender.

Add the cauliflower and beans, then cover and simmer for 10 minutes, or until the vegetables are cooked and most of the liquid has been absorbed. Remove the lid and simmer for a few minutes if there is still too much liquid remaining.

Divide the curry among the serving bowls and top with basil and coriander leaves. Serve with basmati rice.

nutrition per serve: Energy 1406 kJ (336 Cal); Fat 5.8 g; Saturated fat 0.7 g; Protein 19.3 g; Carbohydrate 45.6 g; Fibre 14.2 g; Cholesterol 0 mg

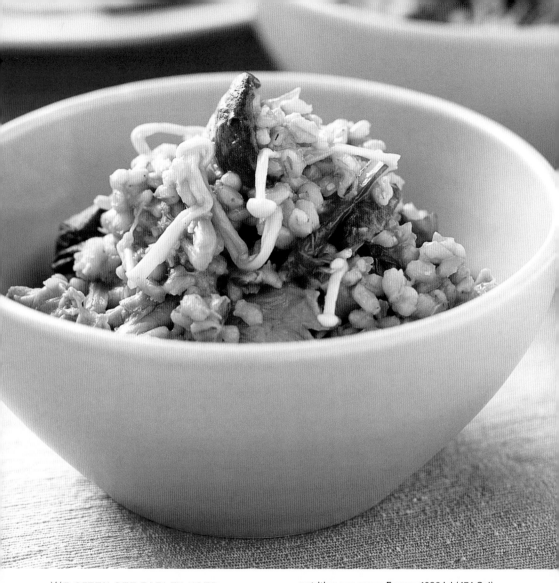

WE OFTEN SEE BARLEY USED
IN HEARTY SOUPS, BUT HERE
IT'S USED INSTEAD OF RICE IN
A PILAFF. BARLEY IS A VERY
LOW-GI FOOD AND A GREAT
SOURCE OF SOLUBLE FIBRE.

nutrition per serve: Energy 1986 kJ (474 Cal)

Fat 13.3 g

Saturated fat 1.9 g

Protein 13.4 g

Carbohydrate 59.4 g

Fibre 16.9 g

Cholesterol 0 mg

PEARL BARLEY AND ASIAN MUSHROOM PILAFF

330 g (11½ oz/1½ cups) pearl barley
3 dried shiitake mushrooms
625 ml (21½ fl oz/2½ cups) vegetable stock
125 ml (4 fl oz/½ cup) dry sherry
2 tbsp olive oil
1 large onion, finely chopped
3 garlic cloves, crushed
2 tbsp grated fresh ginger
1 tsp sichuan peppercorns, crushed
500 g (1 lb 2 oz) mixed fresh Asian
    mushrooms (oyster, Swiss brown, enoki)

500 g (1 lb 2 oz) choy sum (Chinese
    flowering cabbage), cut into short
    lengths
3 tsp kecap manis
1 tsp sesame oil

PREP TIME: 20 MINUTES + OVERNIGHT
    SOAKING
COOKING TIME: 45 MINUTES
SERVES 4

Soak the barley in enough cold water to cover for at least 6 hours, or preferably overnight. Drain. Soak the shiitake mushrooms in enough boiling water to cover for 15 minutes. Strain, reserving 125 ml (4 fl oz/½ cup) of the soaking liquid. Discard the stalks and thinly slice the mushroom caps.

Heat the stock and sherry in a small saucepan. Cover and keep at a low simmer.

Heat the oil in a large saucepan over medium heat and cook the onion for 4–5 minutes, or until softened. Add the garlic, ginger and peppercorns and cook for 1 minute. Slice the Asian mushrooms, reserving the enoki, if using, for later. Increase the heat, add the mushrooms and cook for 5 minutes, or until softened. Add the barley, shiitake, reserved soaking liquid and hot stock and stir to combine. Bring to the boil, then reduce the heat to low and simmer, covered, for 35 minutes, or until the liquid evaporates.

Steam the choy sum until just wilted. Add the choy sum to the barley mixture along with the enoki mushrooms. Stir in the kecap manis and sesame oil and serve hot.

TOFU BURGER WITH VEGETABLES

FLAVOURSOME, FILLING AND NUTRITIOUS, THIS BURGER CONTAINS FIBRE, CARBOHYDRATE, FOLATE, VITAMIN C, IRON AND CALCIUM.

15 g (½ oz) dried porcini mushrooms

2 red capsicums (peppers), quartered

750 g (1 lb 10 oz) kipfler (fingerling) potatoes, cut into 2 cm (¾ in) slices on the diagonal

olive oil spray

2 red onions, finely chopped

6 garlic cloves, crushed

400 g (14 oz) Swiss brown mushrooms, finely chopped

2 tbsp shredded basil

3 tbsp finely chopped parsley

2 tbsp finely chopped oregano

125 ml (4 fl oz/½ cup) vegetable stock

500 g (1 lb 2 oz) firm tofu, finely grated

200 g (7 oz/2½ cups) fresh wholegrain breadcrumbs

1 egg, lightly beaten

4 round wholegrain rolls or buns

2 handfuls baby rocket (arugula) leaves

160 g (5½ oz/⅔ cup) tomato relish

PREP TIME: 25 MINUTES + 20 MINUTES
SOAKING + 2 HOURS REFRIGERATION

COOKING TIME: 1¼ HOURS

SERVES 4

Preheat the oven to 200°C (400°F/Gas 6). Put the porcini in a bowl, cover with boiling water and set aside for 20 minutes. Drain, squeeze out excess moisture and finely chop. Put the capsicum under a preheated grill (broiler), skin side up, and cook for 10 minutes, or until the skin blackens and blisters. Put in a plastic bag to cool, then peel off the skin.

Put the potatoes in a baking dish, spray with oil and toss to coat. Sprinkle with sea salt and bake for 45 minutes, turning halfway through, or until golden.

Spray a non-stick frying pan with oil and heat over high heat. Cook the onion for 3 minutes, then add the garlic, Swiss brown and porcini mushrooms and cook for 3 minutes. Stir in the herbs, then add the stock and cook, stirring, for 4–5 minutes, or until the liquid has evaporated. Cool, then transfer to a bowl and stir in the tofu, 40 g (1½ oz/½ cup) of the breadcrumbs and egg until combined. Season with salt and pepper. Refrigerate for 2 hours.

Divide the tofu mixture into four patties and coat in the remaining breadcrumbs. Spray a non-stick pan with oil and heat over high heat. Cook the patties for 4–5 minutes on each side, or until golden.

Halve the rolls and toast them. Arrange the rocket, patties and capsicum on each base. Top with the relish, season and top with the remaining bread. Serve with the potatoes.

nutrition per serve: Energy 2804 kJ (670 Cal); Fat 15 g; Saturated fat 2.2 g; Protein 37 g; Carbohydrate 87.5 g; Fibre 14.5 g; Cholesterol 47 mg

SPINACH AND RICOTTA CANNELLONI

THIS FAMILY FAVOURITE IS SUITABLE AS AN ENTRÉE OR MAIN MEAL. IT PROVIDES GOOD AMOUNTS OF CALCIUM, FOLATE AND BETA-CAROTENE.

1 tbsp olive oil

2 large onions, chopped

4 garlic cloves, crushed

1 kg (2 lb 4 oz) English spinach, washed, finely chopped

650 g (1 lb 7 oz/2⅔ cups) low-fat ricotta cheese

2 eggs, lightly beaten

pinch of freshly grated nutmeg

olive oil spray

2 x 400 g (14 oz) tins chopped tomatoes

125 ml (4 fl oz/½ cup) dry white wine

2 tbsp tomato paste (concentrated purée)

1 tsp soft brown sugar

2 tbsp chopped basil

250 g (9 oz) dried cannelloni tubes

110 g (3¾ oz/¾ cup) grated reduced-fat mozzarella cheese

35 g (1¼ oz/⅓ cup) grated parmesan cheese

PREP TIME: 45 MINUTES

COOKING TIME: 1½ HOURS

SERVES 6

Heat 2 teaspoons of the oil in a large saucepan. Add half the onion and cook for 3 minutes, then stir in half the garlic and cook for 1 minute. Add the chopped spinach and cook for 2 minutes. Cover the pan and steam the spinach for 1–2 minutes, or until wilted. Set aside to cool slightly. Transfer to a colander and squeeze to remove the moisture.

Mix the spinach with the ricotta, eggs and nutmeg. Season with salt and freshly ground black pepper. Preheat the oven to 180°C (350°F/Gas 4) and spray a large 35 x 24 x 5 cm (14 x 9½ x 2 in) ovenproof dish with oil.

To make the sauce, heat the remaining oil in a large frying pan and cook the remaining onion over low heat for 5 minutes, then add the remaining garlic and cook for 1 minute. Add the tomatoes, wine, tomato paste, sugar and basil. Bring to the boil, then reduce the heat and simmer for 30 minutes.

Spread one-third of the tomato sauce in the dish. Spoon 2–3 tablespoons of the spinach mixture into each cannelloni tube and arrange neatly in the dish. Spoon the remaining sauce over the top and sprinkle with mozzarella and parmesan. Bake for 40–45 minutes, or until the cannelloni is tender and the top is crisp and golden. Serve with a green salad.

nutrition per serve: Energy 2008 kJ (480 Cal); Fat 16.4 g; Saturated fat 6.3 g; Protein 31.2 g; Carbohydrate 43.5 g; Fibre 9 g; Cholesterol 82 mg

147

VEGETABLE TAGINE WITH COUSCOUS

4 ripe tomatoes

¼ tsp saffron threads

2 tbsp flaked almonds

2 tbsp olive oil

2 onions, thinly sliced

3 garlic cloves, crushed

2 thin carrots, cut into 5 mm (¼ in) slices

1 cinnamon stick

2 tsp ground cumin

1 tsp ground ginger

½ tsp ground turmeric

½ tsp cayenne pepper

300 g (10½ oz) peeled pumpkin (winter squash), cut into 2 cm (¾ in) cubes

400 g (14 oz) tin chickpeas, drained and rinsed

500 ml (17 fl oz/2 cups) vegetable stock

1 zucchini (courgette), halved lengthways, then cut into 1 cm (½ in) slices

4 tbsp raisins

50 g (1¾ oz/½ bunch) coriander (cilantro) leaves, roughly chopped

COUSCOUS

625 ml (21½ fl oz/2½ cups) vegetable stock

465 g (1 lb/2½ cups) couscous

2 tsp reduced-fat margarine

PREP TIME: 25 MINUTES

COOKING TIME: 50 MINUTES

SERVES 6

To peel the tomatoes, score a cross in the base of each tomato. Put in a heatproof bowl and cover with boiling water. Leave for 30 seconds, then transfer to cold water and peel the skin away from the cross. To seed, cut the tomatoes in half and scoop out the seeds with a teaspoon. Cut the tomatoes into quarters.

Dry-fry the saffron threads in a small frying pan over low heat for 1 minute, until darkened. Remove from the heat and cool. Repeat with the almonds, then remove and set aside.

Heat the oil in a large flameproof casserole dish. Add the onion, garlic, carrot, cinnamon stick, cumin, ginger, turmeric, cayenne pepper and saffron. Cook over medium–low heat, stirring often, for 10 minutes. Add the tomatoes, pumpkin and chickpeas and stir to coat. Add the stock and bring to the boil. Cover and simmer for 10 minutes. Stir in the zucchini, raisins and half the coriander. Cover and simmer for a further 20 minutes.

To make the couscous, bring the stock to the boil in a large saucepan. Put the couscous in a large heatproof bowl and pour over the hot stock. Cover and leave for 5 minutes, then fluff the grains with a fork. Stir in the margarine and season.

Spoon the couscous into serving bowls. Spoon the vegetables and sauce on top and sprinkle with the toasted almonds and the remaining coriander. Serve at once.

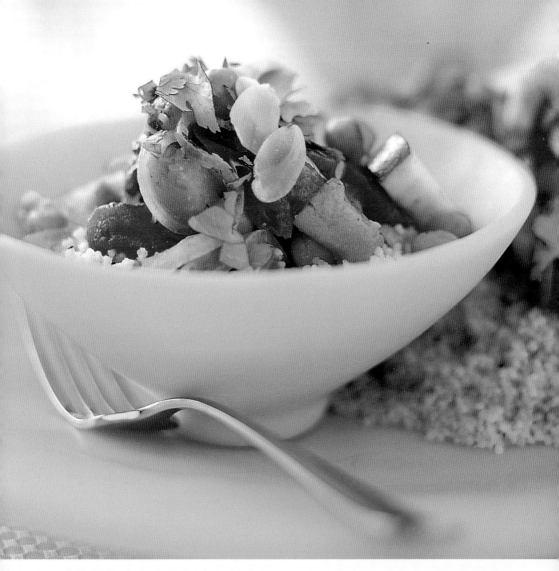

THIS COLOURFUL TAGINE CONTAINS
AN ARRAY OF VEGETABLES AND IS
AN EXCELLENT SOURCE OF BETA-
CAROTENE—AN ANTIOXIDANT
THAT'S GOOD FOR THE HEART AND
EYES. THE SPICES ADD AROMA,
FLAVOUR AND EXTRA MINERALS.

nutrition per serve: Energy 2149 kJ (513 Cal)
Fat 11.3 g
Saturated fat 1.7 g
Protein 16.8 g
Carbohydrate 82.3 g
Fibre 7.1 g
Cholesterol 0 mg

RED LENTIL PILAFF WITH GREEN VEGETABLES

THIS LOW-GI, LOW-FAT DISH PROVIDES LARGE AMOUNTS OF MOST VITAMINS, MINERALS AND OTHER HEALTHY PLANT COMPOUNDS NECESSARY FOR MAINTAINING GOOD HEALTH.

750 ml (26 fl oz/3 cups) vegetable stock
1 tbsp olive oil
1 onion, chopped
3 garlic cloves, chopped
3 tsp garam masala
200 g (7 oz/1 cup) basmati rice
200 g (7 oz/1 cup) red lentils
220 g (7¾ oz) broccolini, cut into 5 cm (2 in) lengths

100 g (3½ oz) snow peas (mangetout), trimmed
thinly sliced spring onions (scallions), to garnish

PREP TIME: 20 MINUTES
COOKING TIME: 30 MINUTES
SERVES 4–6

Bring the stock to the boil in a saucepan, then reduce the heat to a low simmer.

Heat the oil in a large saucepan and add the onion, garlic and garam masala. Cook over medium heat for 3 minutes, or until soft. Stir in the rice and lentils and cook for 2 minutes. Add the hot stock and stir well. Slowly bring to the boil, then reduce the heat and simmer, covered, for 15–20 minutes, or until the rice and lentils are cooked and all the stock has been absorbed. Gently fluff the rice with a fork.

Meanwhile, steam the broccolini and snow peas for 2–3 minutes, or until just cooked. Serve at once with the pilaff and garnish with the spring onion.

HINT:
• You can use any green vegetables for this dish—try broccoli, bok choy (pak choy) or Chinese broccoli (gai larn).

nutrition per serve (6): Energy 1179 kJ (282 Cal); Fat 4.5 g; Saturated fat 0.7 g; Protein 13.2 g; Carbohydrate 44.1 g; Fibre 7.6 g; Cholesterol 0 mg

VEGETARIAN CHILLI

BURGHUL AND LEGUMES ARE COMBINED IN THIS DISH TO PRODUCE A VERY
FILLING MEAL, WHICH WILL KEEP YOU GOING FOR HOURS—A GOOD CHOICE
FOR PEOPLE WHO ARE WATCHING THEIR WEIGHT.

130 g (4½ oz/¾ cup) burghul (bulgur)
250 ml (9 fl oz/1 cup) hot water
2 tsp olive oil
1 large onion, finely chopped
2 garlic cloves, crushed
1 tsp chilli powder
2 tsp ground cumin
1 tsp cayenne pepper
½ tsp ground cinnamon
2 x 400 g (14 oz) tins chopped tomatoes
750 ml (26 fl oz/3 cups) reduced-salt
    vegetable stock

2 x 400 g (14 oz) tins red kidney beans,
    drained and rinsed
2 x 300 g (10½ oz) tins chickpeas, drained
    and rinsed
310 g (11 oz) tin corn kernels, drained
2 tbsp tomato paste (concentrated purée)
3 tbsp chopped parsley

PREP TIME: 10 MINUTES + 10 MINUTES
    SOAKING
COOKING TIME: 40 MINUTES
SERVES 4

Put the burghul in a bowl, cover with the hot water and soak for 10 minutes.

Heat the oil in a large saucepan over medium heat and cook the onion for 10 minutes,
stirring often, until soft and golden. Add the garlic, chilli powder, cumin, cayenne pepper
and cinnamon and cook, stirring, for a further minute.

Add the tomatoes, stock and burghul. Bring to the boil, then reduce the heat and simmer
for 10 minutes. Stir in the kidney beans, chickpeas, corn and tomato paste and simmer for
20 minutes, stirring often. Garnish with the parsley. If desired, top with a little low-fat plain
yoghurt or sour cream, or grated low-fat cheddar cheese.

HINTS:
• Chilli will keep for up to 3 days in the refrigerator and can be frozen for up to 1 month.
• Substitute the burghul with brown basmati rice if you prefer.

nutrition per serve: Energy 2086 kJ (498 Cal); Fat 7.2 g; Saturated fat 1.1 g; Protein 22.7 g;
Carbohydrate 72.3 g; Fibre 24.4 g; Cholesterol 0 mg

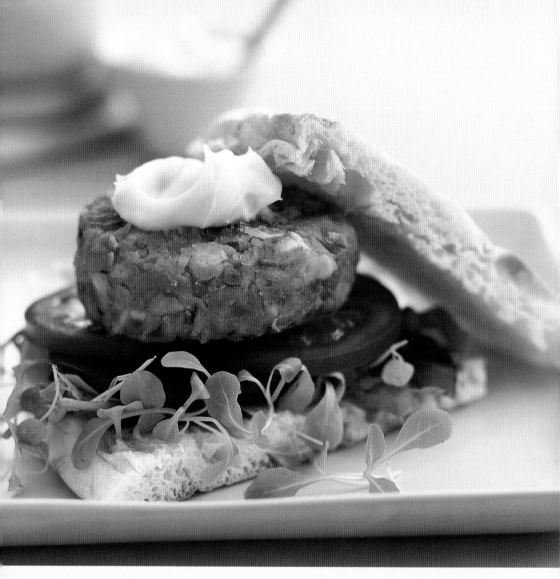

THESE HEALTHY BEAN BURGERS
ARE A VERY FILLING HIGH-FIBRE
VEGETARIAN MEAL. THIS DISH
ALSO PROVIDES FOLATE,
POTASSIUM AND ANTIOXIDANTS.

nutrition per serve: Energy 1994 kJ (476 Cal)
Fat 6.2 g
Saturated fat 1 g
Protein 18 g
Carbohydrate 81.7 g
Fibre 11.7 g
Cholesterol <1 mg

BEAN BURGERS AND SALAD ON TURKISH BREAD

425 g (15 oz) tin cannellini beans or butter
   beans, drained and rinsed
olive oil spray
1 onion, finely chopped
2 garlic cloves, finely chopped
1 green chilli, seeded and finely chopped
1 tsp ground cumin
1 zucchini (courgette), grated
1 carrot, grated
80 g (2¾ oz/1 cup) fresh wholegrain
   breadcrumbs
2 tsp olive oil

2 handfuls mixed salad leaves
225 g (8 oz) tin sliced beetroot, drained
2 large ripe tomatoes, sliced
1 loaf Turkish pide bread, cut into 4 slices,
   then sliced horizontally
4 tbsp low-fat mayonnaise

PREP TIME: 20 MINUTES + 20 MINUTES
   REFRIGERATION
COOKING TIME: 10 MINUTES
SERVES 4

Mash the beans with a fork and place in a large bowl. Spray a heavy-based frying pan with the oil. Add the onion, garlic and chilli and cook for 3 minutes, or until softened. Stir in the cumin and transfer the onion mixture to the bowl with the beans.

Add the grated zucchini, carrot and breadcrumbs to the bowl. Use clean hands to mix the ingredients. Form into four balls, then flatten to 10 cm (4 in) patties. Cover and refrigerate for at least 20 minutes.

Heat a heavy-based non-stick frying pan over medium heat and add the olive oil. Cook the patties over medium heat for 2–3 minutes on each side, or until golden and heated through. Spray each side of the patties with oil as you cook them.

To serve, arrange the salad leaves, beetroot and tomato slices on each bread base. Add a bean patty, some mayonnaise and place the remaining bread half on top.

HINT:
• For variation, top the patties with some tomato relish or chutney.

PUMPKIN AND BROAD BEAN RISOTTO

RISOTTOS ARE GREAT FOR WEEKNIGHT DINNERS, AND YOU CAN VARY THE BASIC RECIPE BY ADDING WHATEVER VEGETABLES YOU HAVE ON HAND—USE PEAS INSTEAD OF BROAD BEANS OR SWEET POTATO INSTEAD OF PUMPKIN.

350 g (12 oz) peeled pumpkin (winter squash)
olive oil spray
750 ml (26 fl oz/3 cups) vegetable stock
1 tbsp olive oil
1 large onion, finely chopped
2 garlic cloves, finely chopped
220 g (7¾ oz/1 cup) arborio rice
200 g (7 oz) Swiss brown mushrooms, halved

310 g (11 oz/2 cups) frozen broad (fava) beans, thawed, peeled
4 tbsp grated parmesan cheese

PREP TIME: 35 MINUTES
COOKING TIME: 1 HOUR
SERVES 4

Preheat the oven to 200°C (400°F/Gas 6). Cut the pumpkin into small chunks, put in a roasting tin and spray lightly with oil. Bake, turning occasionally, for 20 minutes, or until tender. Cover and set aside.

Put the stock in a saucepan, bring to the boil, then reduce the heat to low and keep at simmering point.

Heat the oil in a large heavy-based frying pan. Add the onion and garlic, cover and cook for 10 minutes over low heat. Add the rice and cook, stirring, for 2 minutes. Gradually stir in 125 ml (4 fl oz/½ cup) of the hot stock and continue to stir the rice until the stock has been absorbed. Stir in another 125 ml (4 fl oz/½ cup) of hot stock. When the stock is absorbed, add the mushrooms and continue adding the remaining stock, a little at a time, until all the stock is absorbed and the rice is just tender—this will take about 20 minutes.

Stir in the pumpkin and broad beans to heat through. Divide the risotto among serving bowls, season with freshly ground black pepper and sprinkle with grated parmesan.

nutrition per serve: Energy 1716 kJ (410 Cal); Fat 9.4 g; Saturated fat 2.7 g; Protein 16.4 g; Carbohydrate 61.1 g; Fibre 7.1 g; Cholesterol 6 mg

TEMPEH STIR-FRY

THIS IS A GREAT VEGETARIAN DISH BECAUSE IT PROVIDES PROTEIN AND MANY VITAMINS AND MINERALS. TEMPEH IS SOLD IN HEALTH FOOD SHOPS AND SUPERMARKETS, AND IS AVAILABLE EITHER PLAIN OR FLAVOURED.

400 g (14 oz/2 cups) basmati rice, rinsed and drained
1 tsp sesame oil
2 tsp peanut oil
2 garlic cloves, crushed
1 tbsp grated fresh ginger
1 red chilli, thinly sliced
4 spring onions (scallions), sliced on the diagonal
300 g (10½ oz) tempeh, diced
500 g (1 lb 2 oz) baby bok choy (pak choy) leaves

800 g (1 lb 12 oz/1 bunch) Chinese broccoli (gai larn), chopped
125 ml (4 fl oz/½ cup) mushroom oyster sauce
2 tbsp rice vinegar
2 tbsp chopped coriander (cilantro) leaves
40 g (1½ oz/¼ cup) cashew nuts, toasted

PREP TIME: 15 MINUTES
COOKING TIME: 30 MINUTES
SERVES 4

Put the rice and 1 litre (35 fl oz/4 cups) water in a saucepan and bring to the boil over medium heat. Reduce the heat to low, cover and cook for 20 minutes, or until the rice is tender. Remove from the heat and set aside, covered, for 5 minutes.

Meanwhile, heat a wok until very hot, add the sesame and peanut oils and swirl to coat. Reduce the heat to medium, add the garlic, ginger, chilli and spring onion and cook for 1–2 minutes, or until the spring onion is soft. Add the tempeh and cook for 5 minutes, or until golden. Remove from the wok and keep warm.

Add half the bok choy, half the Chinese broccoli and 1 tablespoon water to the wok and cook, covered, for 3–4 minutes, or until the greens are wilted. Remove and repeat with the remaining greens and more water.

Return the greens and tempeh to the wok, add the mushroom oyster sauce and vinegar and warm through. Top with the coriander and nuts and serve with the rice.

HINT:
• You can add lentils or chickpeas to the rice to add more protein.

nutrition per serve: Energy 2917 kJ (697 Cal); Fat 17.9 g; Saturated fat 3.3 g; Protein 29.6 g; Carbohydrate 100.3 g; Fibre 14.4 g; Cholesterol 0 mg

VEGETARIAN PAELLA

200 g (7 oz/1 cup) dried haricot (navy) beans
¼ tsp saffron threads
2 tbsp olive oil
1 onion, diced
1 red capsicum (pepper), thinly sliced
5 garlic cloves, crushed
275 g (9¾ oz/1¼ cups) paella or arborio rice
1 tbsp sweet paprika
½ tsp mixed (pumpkin pie) spice
750 ml (26 fl oz/3 cups) vegetable stock
400 g (14 oz) tin diced tomatoes

1½ tbsp tomato paste (concentrated purée)
150 g (5½ oz/1 cup) tinned or frozen soya beans
100 g (3½ oz) silverbeet (Swiss chard) leaves (no stems), shredded
400 g (14 oz) tin artichoke hearts, drained and quartered
4 tbsp chopped coriander (cilantro) leaves

PREP TIME: 20 MINUTES + OVERNIGHT SOAKING
COOKING TIME: 40 MINUTES
SERVES 6

Put the haricot beans in a bowl, cover with cold water and leave to soak overnight. Drain and rinse well.

Put the saffron threads in a small frying pan over medium–low heat. Dry-fry, shaking the pan, for 1 minute, or until darkened. Remove from the heat and when cool, crumble into a small bowl. Pour in 125 ml (4 fl oz/½ cup) warm water and set aside to steep.

Heat the oil in a large paella pan or frying pan. Add the onion and capsicum and cook over medium–high heat for 5 minutes, or until the onion softens. Stir in the garlic and cook for 1 minute. Reduce the heat and add the drained beans, rice, paprika, mixed spice and ½ teaspoon salt. Stir to coat. Add the saffron water, stock, tomatoes and tomato paste and bring to the boil. Cover, reduce the heat and simmer for 20 minutes.

Stir in the soya beans, silverbeet and artichoke hearts and cook, covered, for 8 minutes, or until all the liquid has been absorbed and the rice and beans are tender. Turn off the heat and leave for 5 minutes. Stir in the coriander just before serving.

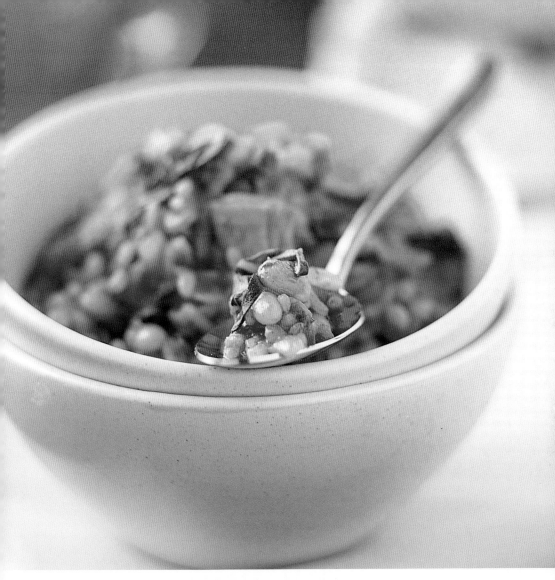

THIS HEARTY AND NUTRITIOUS
HIGH-FIBRE DISH IS RICH IN
POTASSIUM AND ANTIOXIDANTS.
TOP WITH SOME LOW-FAT
YOGHURT OR SOUR CREAM FOR
EXTRA CALCIUM, AND SERVE AS
A SIDE DISH OR A MAIN MEAL.

nutrition per serve: Energy 1661 kJ (397 Cal)
Fat 9.4 g
Saturated fat 1.4 g
Protein 15.6 g
Carbohydrate 57.6 g
Fibre 12 g
Cholesterol 0 mg

157

ASIAN GREENS WITH ROASTED CASHEWS

SERVE THIS EITHER AS A SIDE DISH, WITH A BOWL OF BROWN RICE FOR A SIMPLE MEAL OR WITH THE SPICED LENTIL AND RICE PILAFF ON PAGE 139. THIS DISH IS AN EXCELLENT SOURCE OF FOLATE AND ANTIOXIDANTS.

40 g (1½ oz/¼ cup) cashew nuts
¼ tsp sesame seeds
300 g (10½ oz) broccoli, cut into florets
500 g (1 lb 2 oz) baby bok choy (pak choy), leaves separated
150 g (5½ oz) snow peas (mangetout)
150 g (5½ oz) asparagus spears, halved on the diagonal
1 tbsp peanut oil

2 tsp sesame oil
2 tbsp kecap manis
2 tsp mushroom soy sauce

PREP TIME: 10 MINUTES

COOKING TIME: 10 MINUTES

SERVES 4

Put the cashew nuts in a small frying pan and dry-fry for 1 minute, or until light golden. Remove from the pan. When cool, roughly chop and put into a bowl. Add the sesame seeds to the pan and dry-fry until light golden, then remove to the bowl with the cashews.

Steam the green vegetables for 3–4 minutes, or until just tender.

Heat the peanut and sesame oils in a small wok or saucepan. Add the kecap manis and mushroom soy sauce and cook, stirring, over medium heat for 1 minute, or until heated through. Add the vegetables to the wok and briefly toss to heat through. Sprinkle with the cashew nuts and sesame seeds.

nutrition per serve: Energy 817 kJ (195 Cal); Fat 12.5 g; Saturated fat 2 g; Protein 9.1 g; Carbohydrate 8.8 g; Fibre 6.8 g; Cholesterol 0 mg

STUFFED EGGPLANTS

THIS IS AN EXCELLENT MEAL FOR VEGETARIANS, WITH SLOWLY DIGESTED
CARBOHYDRATE, PROTEIN, VITAMIN C, B VITAMINS AND ANTIOXIDANTS.

60 g (2¼ oz/⅓ cup) brown lentils

2 large eggplants (aubergines)

olive oil spray

1 red onion, chopped

2 garlic cloves, crushed

1 red capsicum (pepper), finely chopped

40 g (1½ oz/¼ cup) pine nuts, toasted

440 g (15½ oz) tin chopped tomatoes

140 g (5 oz/¾ cup) cooked short-grain
  brown rice

2 tbsp chopped coriander (cilantro) leaves

1 tbsp chopped parsley

2 tbsp grated parmesan cheese

PREP TIME: 20 MINUTES

COOKING TIME: 1 HOUR

SERVES 4

Put the lentils in a saucepan, cover with water and simmer for 25 minutes, or until soft.
Drain and set aside.

Slice the eggplants in half lengthways and scoop out the flesh, leaving a 1 cm (½ in) thick
shell. Chop the flesh finely.

Spray a deep, large non-stick frying pan with the oil, add 1 tablespoon water to the pan,
then add the onion and garlic and stir over medium heat until softened. Add the lentils,
capsicum, pine nuts, tomatoes, rice and eggplant flesh and stir over medium heat for
10 minutes, or until the eggplant has softened. Add the coriander and parsley. Season,
then toss until well mixed.

Cook the eggplant shells in boiling water for 4–5 minutes, or until tender. Spoon the filling
into the shells and sprinkle with the parmesan. Place under a preheated grill (broiler) and
cook for 5–10 minutes, or until golden. Serve immediately.

nutrition per serve: Energy 1100 kJ (263 Cal); Fat 10.7 g; Saturated fat 1.4 g; Protein 10.8 g;
Carbohydrate 27.1 g; Fibre 8.8 g; Cholesterol 3 mg

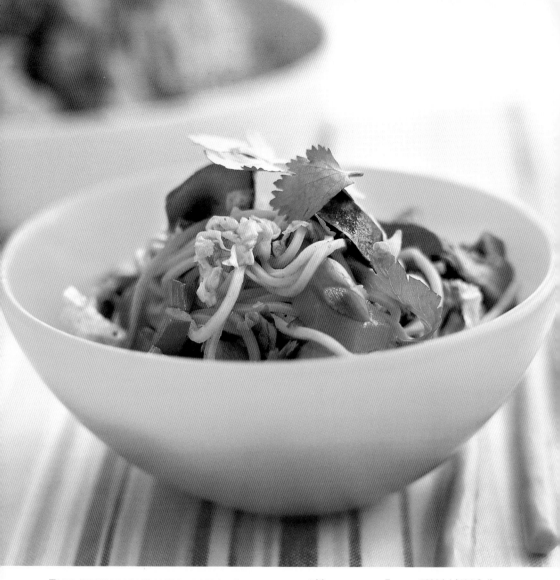

This tasty light meal, with its distinctive Asian flavours, is quick and easy to make for a weeknight meal. It's also rich in various antioxidants, folate and potassium.

nutrition per serve: Energy 1692 kJ (404 Cal)
Fat 9.6 g
Saturated fat 1.2 g
Protein 23.3 g
Carbohydrate 46.3 g
Fibre 11.4 g
Cholesterol 9 mg

VEGETABLE STIR-FRY WITH EGG NOODLES

200 g (7 oz) dried egg noodles

2 tsp canola oil

8 spring onions (scallions), cut into 2.5 cm (1 in) lengths

3 cm (1¼ in) square piece fresh ginger, cut into thin matchsticks

2 garlic cloves, crushed

200 g (7 oz) Swiss brown mushrooms, quartered

1 red capsicum (pepper), thinly sliced

1 zucchini (courgette), cut on the diagonal into 1 cm (½ in) slices

1 carrot, thinly sliced on the diagonal

300 g (10½ oz) broccoli florets

300 g (10½ oz) Chinese cabbage (wong bok), shredded

2 tbsp hoisin sauce

3 tbsp sake or dry sherry

300 g (10½ oz) packet firm tofu, drained and cut into cubes

1 handful coriander (cilantro) leaves, plus extra, to serve

PREP TIME: 20 MINUTES

COOKING TIME: 15 MINUTES

SERVES 4

Bring a large saucepan of water to the boil. Add the noodles and cook for 5 minutes, or until tender. Drain.

Heat a wok over high heat, add the oil and swirl to coat. Add the spring onion and ginger to the wok and stir-fry for 1 minute. Add the garlic and mushrooms and cook for 1 minute, then add the capsicum, zucchini, carrot and broccoli and stir-fry for 3–4 minutes. Pour in 1–2 tablespoons water to help steam the vegetables, if necessary. Add the cabbage, hoisin sauce and sake and stir-fry for 2–3 minutes, or until the cabbage has wilted and all the ingredients are well combined.

Toss in the tofu, noodles and coriander and gently stir until well coated in the sauce. Serve immediately sprinkled with extra coriander leaves.

SWEET THINGS

CREPES WITH WARM FRUIT COMPOTE

This delicious fruit compote makes a great dessert served with crepes, or you can enjoy the compote with a dollop of plain or vanilla yoghurt.

CREPES
60 g (2¼ oz/½ cup) plain (all-purpose) flour
2 eggs
250 ml (9 fl oz/1 cup) skim milk
canola oil spray
2 tsp caster (superfine) sugar

COMPOTE
100 g (3½ oz) whole dried apricots
3 tbsp port or Muscat, or use orange juice

1 vanilla bean, halved lengthways
2 firm pears, peeled, cored and quartered
2 cinnamon sticks
425 g (15 oz) tin pitted prunes in syrup, drained, syrup reserved

Prep time: 20 minutes + 30 minutes resting
Cooking time: 20 minutes
Serves 4

Put the flour in a bowl and gradually add the combined eggs and milk, whisking to remove any lumps. Cover the batter with plastic wrap and set aside for 30 minutes.

Meanwhile, to make the compote, put the apricots and port in a saucepan and cook, covered, over low heat for 2–3 minutes, or until softened. Scrape the seeds from the vanilla bean and add the bean and seeds to the pan along with the pear, cinnamon sticks and prune syrup. Simmer, covered, stirring occasionally, for 4 minutes, or until the pear has softened. Add the prunes and simmer for 1 minute.

Heat a 20 cm (8 in) non-stick crepe pan or frying pan over medium heat. Lightly spray with oil. Pour 3 tablespoons of the batter into the pan and swirl evenly over the base. Cook each crepe for 1 minute, or until the underside is golden. Turn it over and cook the other side for 30 seconds, then remove. Keep warm and repeat to make eight crepes in total.

Fold the crepes into triangles and sprinkle with the sugar. Serve with the compote.

nutrition per serve: Energy 1350 kJ (323 Cal); Fat 4.1 g; Saturated fat 0.9 g; Protein 9.2 g; Carbohydrate 56.4 g; Fibre 6.3 g; Cholesterol 96 mg

STEWED PEAR, APPLE AND RHUBARB WITH CUSTARD

DESSERTS BASED ON FRESH FRUIT ARE GOOD CHOICES WHEN YOU'RE TRYING TO EAT A HEALTHY DIET BECAUSE THEY PROVIDE FIBRE, VITAMINS AND MINERALS, MAKING THEM A QUALITY TREAT.

2 tbsp blackcurrant syrup
2 large pears, peeled, cored and quartered
1 large apple, peeled, cored and quartered
500 g (1 lb 2 oz) rhubarb, trimmed, cut into
  3 cm (1¼ in) pieces
500 ml (17 fl oz/2 cups) skim milk
60 g (2¼ oz/¼ cup) caster (superfine) sugar
1½ tbsp custard powder

PREP TIME: 20 MINUTES
COOKING TIME: 20 MINUTES
SERVES 4

Put the syrup, pears, apple and 3 tablespoons water in a large saucepan and stir to coat the fruit. Cook, covered, over low heat for 4 minutes (keep the heat low or the fruit will scorch on the base of the pan). Add the rhubarb, toss well to combine, then cover and cook for a further 6–7 minutes, or until the fruit is just tender. Remove from the heat, cover and set aside.

Put the milk and sugar in a saucepan. Bring to the boil, then reduce the heat and simmer for 3 minutes. Mix the custard powder with 1 tablespoon water and mix to a smooth paste. Return the milk to the boil, stir in the custard powder mixture and whisk constantly until the mixture boils and thickens and coats the back of a wooden spoon.

Place the fruit in serving dishes and drizzle with any liquid from the bottom of the pan. Serve with the warm custard.

HINTS:
• If preferred, the skim milk, sugar and custard powder can be replaced with ready-made low-fat custard.
• Try using your favourite seasonal fruits, such as nectarines or peaches for this dish, cooked until they are just tender.
• Do not overcook the rhubarb or it will fall apart and become stringy.

nutrition per serve: Energy 1034 kJ (247 Cal); Fat 0.6 g; Saturated fat 0.2 g; Protein 6.3 g; Carbohydrate 53.3 g; Fibre 5.1 g; Cholesterol 4 mg

APPLE PIE

PASTRY
canola oil spray
150 g (5½ oz/1 cup) wholemeal
   (whole-wheat) flour
125 g (4½ oz/1 cup) plain (all-purpose) flour
30 g (1 oz/¼ cup) self-raising flour
2 tbsp soft brown sugar
½ tsp ground cinnamon
125 g (4½ oz) reduced-fat margarine,
   chilled and chopped
1 egg yolk
3–4 tbsp chilled water

FILLING
750 g (1 lb 10 oz) granny smith apples,
   peeled, cored and sliced (4 large apples)
2 tbsp soft brown sugar
1 tbsp lemon juice
55 g (2 oz/⅓ cup) chopped pitted dates
40 g (1½ oz/⅓ cup) raisins
30 g (1 oz/¼ cup) chopped walnuts
milk, to brush
demerara (raw) sugar, to sprinkle

PREP TIME: 40 MINUTES + 45 MINUTES
   REFRIGERATION
COOKING TIME: 1 HOUR 5 MINUTES
SERVES 8

Preheat the oven to 180°C (350°F/Gas 4). Lightly spray an 18 cm (7 in) pie dish with oil.

To make the pastry, sift the flours into a food processor bowl and return the husks to the bowl. Add the sugar and cinnamon and briefly pulse. Add the margarine and process for 30 seconds, or until fine and crumbly. Add the egg yolk and 2 tablespoons chilled water and process until the mixture just comes together. Add the remaining water if necessary to form a soft dough. Gently gather the dough together and lift onto a lightly floured work surface. Press into a ball and flatten slightly. Wrap in plastic and refrigerate for 30 minutes.

To make the filling, place the apple slices, brown sugar, lemon juice and 2 tablespoons water in a large saucepan, cover and bring to the boil, then reduce the heat and simmer gently for 15 minutes. Stir in the dried fruit and walnuts, then leave the mixture to cool.

Roll out two-thirds of the pastry between two sheets of baking paper, to fit the dish. Invert the pastry into the dish, allowing any excess to hang over the side, then trim. Cover and refrigerate for 15 minutes. Line the pastry shell with a piece of crumpled baking paper, pour in some baking beads and bake for 10 minutes. Remove the paper and baking beads and bake for a further 10 minutes. Spoon the apple mixture into the pastry shell.

Roll the remaining pastry out to fit the top. Brush the edge of the pastry in the dish with water and place the pastry lid on top. Trim, then press the edges together. Make several slits in the top of the pie, brush with milk and sprinkle over the sugar. Bake for 30 minutes, or until the pastry is crisp and golden. Serve with whipped light cream, if desired.

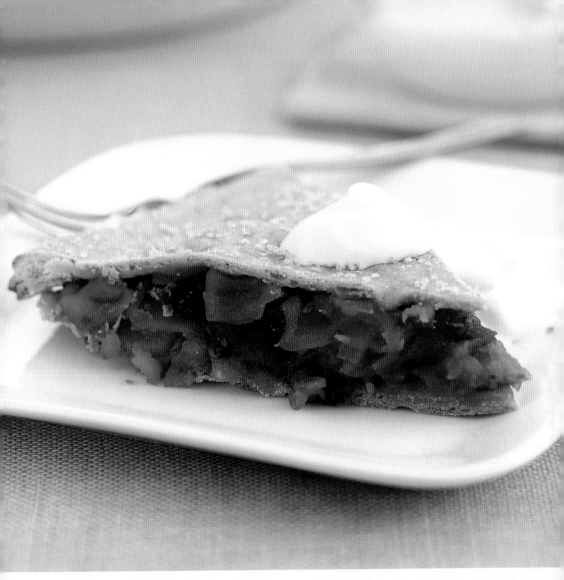

APPLE PIE IS A FAMILY FAVOURITE
AND THIS VERSION IS MADE WITH A
WHOLEMEAL PASTRY. DON'T FORGET
TO ADD SOME STEAM HOLES IN THE
TOP OF THE PIE BEFORE COOKING IT
OR THE PASTRY WILL END UP SOGGY.

nutrition per serve: Energy 1322 kJ (316 Cal)

Fat 9.7 g

Saturated fat 3.1 g

Protein 5.6 g

Carbohydrate 50 g

Fibre 5.6 g

Cholesterol 36 mg

WHOLEMEAL BANANA BREAD

This filling banana bread contains more fibre than the regular version and is just as delicious. Serve warm, cold or toasted, with low-fat yoghurt or fromage frais.

olive oil spray

95 g (3½ oz/½ cup) soft brown sugar

1 egg

250 g (9 oz/1 cup) low-fat vanilla fromage frais

2 tbsp canola oil

235 g (8½ oz/1 cup) mashed banana (2 bananas)

30 g (1 oz/¼ cup) pepitas (pumpkin seeds)

60 g (2¼ oz/½ cup) sultanas (golden raisins)

80 g (2¾ oz/½ cup) stoneground self-raising flour

110 g (3¾ oz/⅔ cup) stoneground wholemeal (whole-wheat) self-raising flour

½ tsp bicarbonate of soda (baking soda)

3 tbsp unprocessed wheat bran

1 tsp ground cinnamon

½ tsp ground nutmeg

Prep time: 15 minutes

Cooking time: 50 minutes

Makes 8 slices

Preheat the oven to 160°C (315°F/Gas 2–3). Spray an 18 x 10 cm (7 x 4 in) loaf (bar) tin with oil and line the base with baking paper.

Put the sugar, egg, fromage frais and oil in a large bowl and whisk until well combined. Stir in the banana, pepitas and sultanas, then fold in the sifted flours (return the husks to the bowl), bicarbonate of soda, bran, cinnamon and nutmeg.

Spoon the mixture into the prepared tin and bake for 50 minutes, or until cooked through when tested with a skewer. Serve warm or cold with low-fat yoghurt or fromage frais.

nutrition per slice: Energy 1175 kJ (281 Cal); Fat 7.7 g; Saturated fat 1 g; Protein 8 g; Carbohydrate 43 g; Fibre 4.3 g; Cholesterol 25 mg

RHUBARB, APPLE AND BARLEY CRUMBLE

TRY THIS NEW VERSION OF TRADITIONAL APPLE CRUMBLE—WITH RHUBARB FOR EXTRA COLOUR AND FLAVOUR, AND ROLLED BARLEY INSTEAD OF OATS FOR MORE FIBRE.

400 g (14 oz/1 bunch) trimmed rhubarb, washed and cut into 3 cm (1¼ in) pieces
1 large green apple, peeled, cored and chopped
2 tbsp soft brown sugar
75 g (2½ oz/¾ cup) wholegrain rolled barley
40 g (1½ oz/¼ cup) stoneground wholemeal (whole-wheat) flour

50 g (1¾ oz/¼ cup) soft brown sugar, extra
30 g (1 oz) reduced-fat margarine
1 tbsp pepitas (pumpkin seeds) or sunflower seeds

PREP TIME: 20 MINUTES + COOLING
COOKING TIME: 30 MINUTES
SERVES 4

Preheat the oven to 180°C (350°F/Gas 4). Put the rhubarb, apple and sugar in a saucepan with 2 tablespoons water. Gently stir to dissolve the sugar. Cover and simmer over low heat for 8–10 minutes, or until the fruit is cooked but not broken up. Pour into a 1.25 litre (44 fl oz/5 cup) ovenproof dish and set aside until completely cool.

Meanwhile, put the rolled barley, flour and extra sugar in a bowl. Rub in the margarine with your fingertips until the mixture is crumbly. Stir in the pepitas.

Sprinkle the crumble over the fruit. Bake for 15–20 minutes, or until the crumble is lightly browned. Serve hot or warm with low-fat yoghurt, custard or ice cream.

HINTS:
• Look for rolled barley in a health food shop if you can't find it in a supermarket, or use wholegrain rolled (porridge) oats.
• We used a bunch of rhubarb that already had its leaves trimmed. If your bunch of rhubarb has leaves, look for one around 700 g (1 lb 9 oz).

nutrition per serve: Energy 1060 kJ (253 Cal); Fat 5.2 g; Saturated fat 0.9 g; Protein 4.6 g; Carbohydrate 47.3 g; Fibre 6 g; Cholesterol 0 mg

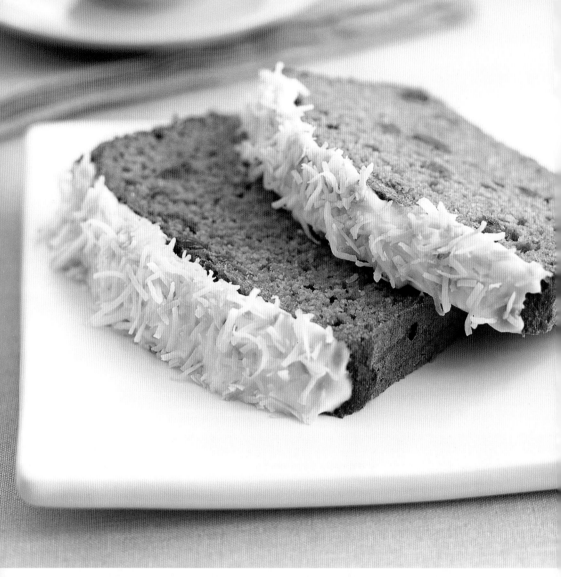

THIS REDUCED-FAT, HIGH-FIBRE VERSION OF CARROT CAKE IS JUST AS TASTY AS THE REGULAR KIND. ADDING FIBRE WILL HELP YOU FEEL SATISFIED AFTER JUST ONE SLICE.

nutrition per slice: Energy 1070 kJ (256 Cal)

Fat 6.4 g

Saturated fat 1.7 g

Protein 7.4 g

Carbohydrate 40 g

Fibre 4.9 g

Cholesterol 32 mg

CARROT CAKE WITH RICOTTA TOPPING

160 g (5½ oz/1 cup) stoneground wholemeal (whole-wheat) self-raising flour

160 g (5½ oz/1 cup) stoneground self-raising flour

1 tsp bicarbonate of soda (baking soda)

2 tsp ground cinnamon

1 tsp mixed (pumpkin pie) spice

75 g (2½ oz/½ cup) unprocessed oat bran

95 g (3½ oz/½ cup) soft brown sugar

60 g (2¼ oz/½ cup) sultanas (golden raisins)

2 eggs, lightly beaten

2 tbsp canola oil

80 ml (2½ fl oz/⅓ cup) skim or no-fat milk

270 g (9½ oz/1 cup) apple purée

300 g (10½ oz) carrots, coarsely grated

RICOTTA TOPPING

185 g (6½ oz/¾ cup) low-fat ricotta cheese

30 g (1 oz/¼ cup) icing (confectioners') sugar

1½ tsp grated lemon zest

15 g (½ oz/¼ cup) shredded coconut, lightly toasted

PREP TIME: 20 MINUTES

COOKING TIME: 1½ HOURS

MAKES 12 SLICES

Preheat the oven to 180°C (350°F/Gas 4). Lightly grease a 21 x 11 cm (8¼ x 4¼ in) loaf (bar) tin and line the base with baking paper.

Sift the flours, bicarbonate of soda and spices into a large bowl. Return the husks to the bowl. Stir in the oat bran, sugar and sultanas. Combine the eggs, oil, milk and apple purée in a large bowl. Stir the egg mixture into the flour mixture, then stir in the carrot.

Spoon into the prepared tin and bake for 1¼ hours, or until a skewer comes out clean and the cake comes away slightly from the sides. Cover with foil if browning too much. Leave for 15 minutes, then turn out onto a wire rack.

To make the ricotta topping, beat the ricotta, icing sugar and lemon zest together until smooth. Spread over the cooled cake and sprinkle over the toasted coconut.

HINT:
• Refrigerate the un-iced cake in an airtight container for up to 5 days. Freeze for up to 1 month.

CHOCOLATE FRUIT AND NUT SLICE

QUICK AND EASY TO MAKE, THIS RECIPE IS GREAT FOR THOSE WHO LOVE TO
ENTERTAIN BUT HAVE LITTLE TIME FOR COOKING. BARLEY MAKES THE SLICE
MORE FILLING, TO HELP YOU FEEL SATISFIED WITH JUST ONE PIECE.

canola oil spray

160 g (5½ oz/1 cup) stoneground
wholemeal (whole-wheat) self-raising
flour

2 tbsp unsweetened cocoa powder

50 g (1¾ oz/½ cup) wholegrain rolled
barley

2 tbsp unprocessed oat bran

35 g (1¼ oz/⅓ cup) ground almonds

30 g (1 oz/⅓ cup) desiccated coconut

60 g (2¼ oz/⅓ cup) soft brown sugar

95 g (3½ oz/½ cup) fruit medley, chopped

60 g (2¼ oz/½ cup) walnuts, chopped

90 g (3¼ oz) reduced-fat margarine, just
melted

1 tbsp pure maple syrup

250 ml (9 fl oz/1 cup) low-fat milk

icing (confectioners') sugar, to dust

PREP TIME: 15 MINUTES

COOKING TIME: 25 MINUTES

MAKES 12 SLICES

Preheat the oven to 180°C (350°F/Gas 4). Spray a 27 x 17 cm (10¾ x 6½ in) shallow
baking tin with oil, then line the base with baking paper, leaving the paper overhanging
the two long sides.

Sift the flour and cocoa into a large bowl, then return any husks to the bowl. Stir in the
rolled barley, oat bran, ground almonds, coconut, brown sugar, fruit medley and walnuts.
Make a well in the centre.

Combine the melted margarine, maple syrup and milk in a small bowl. Add to the flour
mixture and stir until well combined. Spread evenly into the prepared tin.

Bake for 25 minutes, or until cooked and firm. Leave in the tin to cool, then turn out onto
a wire rack to cool completely. Dust with icing sugar and cut into slices. Serve with fresh
berries and low-fat yoghurt or fromage frais, if desired.

HINTS:
• The slice will keep in an airtight container for 5 days. Freeze for up to 1 month.
• Look for rolled barley in health food shops. If you can't find barley, substitute wholegrain
rolled oats.

nutrition per slice: Energy 922 kJ (220 Cal); Fat 10.4 g; Saturated fat 2.5 g; Protein 5 g;
Carbohydrate 26.1 g; Fibre 3.8 g; Cholesterol <1 mg

SUMMER PUDDING

BERRIES NOT ONLY CONTAIN LOTS OF HEALTHY ANTIOXIDANTS, THEY ALSO CONTRIBUTE TO OUR DAILY FIBRE INTAKE, AND THEY TASTE GREAT.

150 g (5½ oz) blackcurrants or blueberries
150 g (5½ oz) redcurrants
150 g (5½ oz) raspberries
150 g (5½ oz) blackberries
200 g (7 oz) strawberries, hulled and
  quartered or halved
125 g (4½ oz/heaped ½ cup) caster
  (superfine) sugar, or to taste

6–8 slices good-quality sliced white bread,
  crusts removed

PREP TIME: 30 MINUTES + OVERNIGHT
  REFRIGERATION
COOKING TIME: 5 MINUTES
SERVES 6

Put all the berries, except the strawberries, in a large saucepan with 125 ml (4 fl oz/½ cup) water and heat gently for 5 minutes, or until the berries begin to soften. Add the strawberries and remove from the heat. Add the sugar, to taste (how much you need will depend on how ripe the fruit is). Set aside to cool.

Line six 170 ml (5½ fl oz/⅔ cup) ovenproof moulds or a 1 litre (35 fl oz/4 cup) pudding basin with the bread. For the small moulds, use one slice of bread for each, cutting a circle of bread to fit the bottom, and strips to fit snugly around the sides. For the basin, cut a large circle out of one slice for the bottom and cut the rest of the bread into wide fingers to fit the side.

Drain a little of the juice off the fruit into a bowl. Dip one side of each piece of bread in the juice before fitting it, juice side down, into the mould, leaving no gaps. Do not squeeze or flatten the bread or it won't absorb the juice.

Fill the centre of each mould with the fruit and pour in a little juice. Cover the tops with the remaining dipped bread, juice side up, and trim to fit. Cover with plastic wrap. For the small moulds sit a small tin, or a similar weight, on top of each. For the basin, place a small plate that fits inside the basin onto the plastic wrap, then weigh it down with a large tin. Place on an oven tray to catch any juices that may overflow and refrigerate overnight. Carefully turn out the pudding and serve with any leftover fruit mixture. Serve with low-fat cream or ice cream, if desired.

HINT:
• You can use any combination of berries to make up a total weight of 800 g (1 lb 12 oz).

nutrition per serve: Energy 884 kJ (211 Cal); Fat 1.1 g; Saturated fat 0.1 g; Protein 4.3 g; Carbohydrate 44.1 g; Fibre 6.8 g; Cholesterol 0 mg

STICKY DATE PUDDING

280 g (10 oz/1²/₃ cups) chopped dates
1 tsp natural vanilla extract
2 tsp bicarbonate of soda (baking soda)
90 g (3¼ oz) reduced-fat margarine
95 g (3½ oz/½ cup) soft brown sugar
2 eggs
150 g (5½ oz/1 cup) wholemeal (whole-
   wheat) self-raising flour
60 g (2¼ oz/½ cup) self-raising flour
2 tbsp unprocessed oat bran

SAUCE
185 ml (6 fl oz/¾ cup) evaporated skim
   milk
95 g (3½ oz/½ cup) soft brown sugar
1 tbsp margarine
1 tsp custard powder

PREP TIME: 15 MINUTES
COOKING TIME: 1 HOUR
SERVES 8

Preheat the oven to 180°C (350°F/Gas 4). Lightly grease and line the base and side of a 20 cm (8 in) round cake tin.

Put the dates and 375 ml (13 fl oz/1½ cups) water in a saucepan. Bring to the boil, then reduce the heat and simmer for 5 minutes, or until soft. Stir in the vanilla and bicarbonate of soda and set aside to cool to room temperature.

Beat the margarine and sugar with electric beaters until pale and creamy. Gradually add the eggs, beating well after each addition—the mixture may look curdled at this stage, but a spoonful of flour will bring it back together. Fold in the sifted flours (return the husks to the bowl), oat bran and the date mixture in two batches, using a metal spoon.

Pour the mixture into the prepared tin. Bake for 50 minutes, or until a skewer comes out clean when inserted into the centre of the pudding. Cool in the tin for 10–15 minutes.

To make the sauce, heat the evaporated milk, sugar and margarine in a saucepan until almost boiling. Combine the custard powder and 1 teaspoon water until smooth, then gradually add to the sauce, stirring continually over medium heat until it thickens slightly. Serve warm with the pudding.

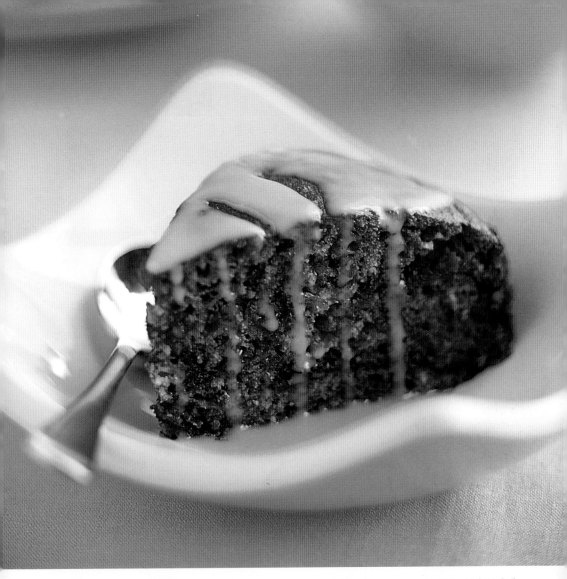

IT'S EASY TO SNEAK SOME FIBRE
INTO CAKES OR BAKED DESSERTS
SUCH AS THIS ONE BY ADDING
ONE OR TWO TABLESPOONS OF
BRAN AND SOME WHOLEMEAL
FLOUR TO THE MIXTURE—NO ONE
WILL NOTICE THE DIFFERENCE.

nutrition per serve: Energy 1599 kJ (382 Cal)
Fat 8.2 g
Saturated fat 1.6 g
Protein 7.8 g
Carbohydrate 67.8 g
Fibre 6.2 g
Cholesterol 48 mg

FIG AND OAT BRAN MUFFINS

ENJOYING SOMETHING SWEET NOW AND THEN CAN MAKE IT EASIER TO STICK WITH A HEALTHY DIET IN THE LONG-TERM. FIGS ARE WONDERFULLY SWEET AND CONTAIN A GOOD AMOUNT OF FIBRE.

125 g (4½ oz/1 cup) self-raising flour
75 g (2½ oz/½ cup) wholemeal (whole-wheat) self-raising flour
½ tsp baking powder
150 g (5½ oz/1 cup) unprocessed oat bran
55 g (2 oz/¼ cup firmly packed) soft brown sugar
250 ml (9 fl oz/1 cup) milk
2 eggs
90 g (3¼ oz/¼ cup) golden syrup or honey

60 g (2¼ oz) unsalted butter, melted and cooled
185 g (6½ oz/1 cup) chopped soft dried figs
3 dried figs, cut into strips, extra

PREP TIME: 15 MINUTES
COOKING TIME: 25 MINUTES
MAKES 12

Preheat the oven to 200°C (400°F/Gas 6). Grease 12 regular muffin holes.

Sift the flours and baking powder into a bowl, return the husks to the bowl, then add the oat bran and sugar. Make a well in the centre.

Combine the milk and eggs in a bowl, whisk together and pour into the well. Add the combined golden syrup and melted butter and fold gently until just combined—the batter should be lumpy. Fold in the chopped figs.

Divide the mixture among the muffin holes and top with the extra strips of fig. Bake for 20–25 minutes, or until the muffins come away from the side of the tin. Cool in the tin for 5 minutes, then transfer to a wire rack.

nutrition per muffin: Energy 1065 kJ (254 Cal); Fat 7 g; Saturated fat 3.7 g; Protein 6.5 g; Carbohydrate 39.3 g; Fibre 6 g; Cholesterol 47 mg

PEAR AND HAZELNUT BRAN MUFFINS

THESE HOME-MADE MUFFINS ARE LOWER IN FAT AND HIGHER IN FIBRE THAN MANY COMMERCIAL VARIETIES. THE HIGHER FIBRE CONTENT AND THE DENSER TEXTURE MAKE JUST ONE MUFFIN A SATISFYING TREAT.

250 g (9 oz) dried pears, chopped
120 g (4¼ oz/2 cups) processed bran cereal
500 ml (17 fl oz/2 cups) reduced-fat milk
310 g (11 oz/1⅓ cups firmly packed) soft
   brown sugar
2 tbsp maple syrup
250 g (9 oz/2 cups) self-raising flour
180 g (6 oz/1¼ cups) hazelnuts, roasted
   and chopped

1 tsp ground cinnamon
1 tsp caster (superfine) sugar

PREP TIME: 10 MINUTES + OVERNIGHT
   REFRIGERATION
COOKING TIME: 25 MINUTES
MAKES 16

Mix the pears, bran cereal, milk, sugar and maple syrup together in a large bowl, then cover and refrigerate overnight.

Preheat the oven to 180°C (350°F/Gas 4). Grease 16 regular muffin holes.

Sift the flour into the pear and bran cereal mixture and add the nuts. Fold gently until just combined—the batter will be lumpy.

Divide the mixture among the muffin holes. Bake for 20–25 minutes, or until the muffins come away from the side of the tin. Cool for 5 minutes, then transfer to a wire rack. Sprinkle with the combined cinnamon and sugar. Serve warm.

nutrition per muffin: Energy 1200 kJ (287 Cal); Fat 8 g; Saturated fat 0.7 g; Protein 5.6 g; Carbohydrate 47 g; Fibre 5.7 g; Cholesterol 2 mg

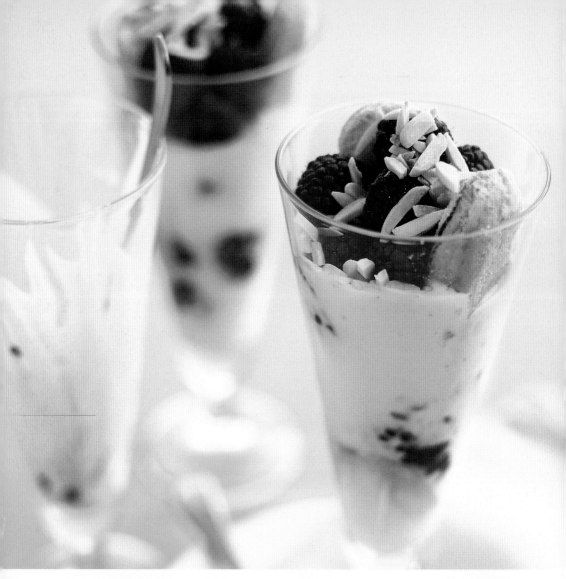

BERRIES AND PASSIONFRUIT
PROVIDE FIBRE, VITAMIN C AND
ANTIOXIDANTS, AND MOST OF THE
FAT IS MONOUNSATURATED FAT.
THIS IS A DELICIOUS, HEALTHY
DESSERT TO SERVE AT YOUR
NEXT CASUAL DINNER PARTY.

nutrition per serve: Energy 1165 kJ (278 Cal)

Fat 7 g

Saturated fat 0.8 g

Protein 13 g

Carbohydrate 34.7 g

Fibre 8.6 g

Cholesterol 38 mg

YOGHURT AND SAVOIARDI PARFAIT

750 g (1 lb 10 oz/3 cups) low-fat plain yoghurt
55 g (2 oz/¼ cup) sugar
10 passionfruit
125 g (4½ oz) savoiardi (sponge finger biscuits), cut to fit parfait glasses
375 g (13 oz/3 cups) fresh or frozen raspberries
60 g (2¼ oz/½ cup) slivered almonds, toasted

PREP TIME: 20 MINUTES + 1 HOUR REFRIGERATION
COOKING TIME: NIL
SERVES 6

Put the yoghurt, sugar and passionfruit pulp in a bowl and mix well to combine. Divide one-third of the mixture among six 250 ml (9 fl oz/1 cup) parfait glasses.

Top the yoghurt mixture with a layer of savoiardi biscuits, then with a layer of raspberries. Repeat with another layer of yoghurt, biscuits and raspberries, and top with a layer of yoghurt. Top with the remaining raspberries and the toasted almonds. Refrigerate for 1 hour before serving.

HINT:
• You can use strawberries instead of raspberries, if you prefer. Hull and slice the strawberries before using.

PRUNE AND CHOC CHIP BISCUITS

QUICK AND EASY TO MAKE, THESE BISCUITS ARE A GREAT TREAT AND THEY
CONTAIN MORE FIBRE THAN MOST COMMERCIAL VARIETIES. ALTHOUGH
THEY'RE LOWER GI, YOU STILL NEED TO EAT THEM IN SENSIBLE AMOUNTS.

**160 g (5½ oz/1 cup) stoneground
  wholemeal (whole-wheat) self-raising
  flour**
**50 g (1¾ oz/½ cup) wholegrain rolled
  barley or oats**
60 g (2¼ oz/⅓ cup) soft brown sugar
30 g (1 oz/⅓ cup) desiccated coconut
2 tbsp unprocessed oat bran
**60 g (2¼ oz/heaped ⅓ cup) dark chocolate
  chips**
**125 g (4½ oz/½ cup) chopped pitted
  prunes**

90 g (3¼ oz) reduced-fat margarine
1 tbsp pure maple syrup
125 ml (4 fl oz/½ cup) buttermilk
2 tsp grated orange zest

PREP TIME: 15 MINUTES
COOKING TIME: 20 MINUTES
MAKES 16

Preheat the oven to 180°C (350°F/Gas 4). Line a baking tray with baking paper.

Sift the flour into a large bowl and return the husks to the bowl. Add the rolled barley, sugar, coconut, oat bran, chocolate chips and prunes. Mix well, separating the prunes with your fingers.

Melt the margarine and maple syrup in a small saucepan over low heat. Add the buttermilk and stir in the orange zest. Pour over the flour mixture and combine until moistened.

Using 1 heaped tablespoon of batter at a time, drop spoonfuls onto the prepared tray, spacing them evenly apart. Bake for 15 minutes, or until golden brown. Leave on the tray for 2–3 minutes, then transfer to a wire rack to cool completely. The biscuits will crisp on cooling.

HINTS:
- Serve with a platter of fresh fruit (berries, stone fruit, citrus fruit, apples and pears) that you can enjoy after you've savoured your portion of 1–2 biscuits.
- Store in an airtight container for up to 1 week.

nutrition per biscuit: Energy 582 kJ (139 Cal); Fat 5.2 g; Saturated fat 2.6 g; Protein 2.5 g; Carbohydrate 20.1 g; Fibre 2.7 g; Cholesterol 1 mg

OAT CRUNCH BISCUITS

THESE OATY BISCUITS ARE MADE WITH APPLE PURÉE TO GIVE THEM FLAVOUR AND SOFTEN THE TEXTURE, WITHOUT ADDING TOO MUCH FAT. THESE ARE HIGHER IN FIBRE THAN MOST COMMERCIAL BISCUITS.

90 g (3¼ oz) unsalted butter, softened
95 g (3½ oz/½ cup) soft brown sugar
1 tsp natural vanilla extract
1 egg
140 g (5 oz) apple purée
200 g (7 oz/2 cups) wholegrain rolled oats
160 g (5½ oz/1 cup) stoneground wholemeal (whole-wheat) self-raising flour
75 g (2½ oz/1 cup) lightly crushed bran flakes

185 g (6½ oz/1 cup) chopped dried apricots
60 g (2¼ oz/½ cup) chopped hazelnuts
30 g (1 oz/¼ cup) pepitas (pumpkin seeds)

PREP TIME: 20 MINUTES
COOKING TIME: 15 MINUTES
MAKES 30

Preheat the oven to 190°C (375°F/Gas 5). Lightly grease two large baking trays.

Using electric beaters, beat the butter and sugar together until creamy, then add the vanilla and egg and beat well. Stir in the apple purée.

Combine the rolled oats, flour, bran flakes, apricots, hazelnuts and pepitas in a large bowl. Stir in the butter mixture until well combined.

Place heaped tablespoons of the mixture on the prepared trays and flatten with a spatula to a rough 7 cm (2¾ in) round. Bake for 12–15 minutes, or until the biscuits are cooked through. Cool on a wire cooling rack, then store in an airtight container.

HINTS:
• Store refrigerated in an airtight container for up to 5 days. You can freeze the biscuits for up to 1 month.
• Combine or replace the chopped apricots with other dried fruits such as dates, prunes or raisins. Replace the hazelnuts with almonds or macadamias.

nutrition per biscuit: Energy 503 kJ (120 Cal); Fat 5.1 g; Saturated fat 1.9 g; Protein 2.6 g; Carbohydrate 14.9 g; Fibre 2.3 g; Cholesterol 14 mg

FRUITY BRAN LOAF

olive oil spray
60 g (2¼ oz/1 cup) processed bran cereal
435 ml (15¼ fl oz/1¾ cups) skim milk
380 g (13½ oz/2 cups) dried fruit medley
95 g (3½ oz/½ cup) soft brown sugar
240 g (8½ oz/1½ cups) stoneground
    wholemeal (whole-wheat) self-raising
    flour
1 tsp ground cinnamon

PREP TIME: 15 MINUTES + 1 HOUR SOAKING
COOKING TIME: 50 MINUTES
MAKES 10 SLICES

Preheat the oven to 180°C (350°F/Gas 4). Spray a 20 x 10 cm (8 x 4 in) loaf (bar) tin with oil and line the base with baking paper.

Put the bran cereal in a large bowl. Stir in the milk, fruit medley and sugar. Set aside for at least 1 hour to soften the bran.

Meanwhile, sift the flour and cinnamon into a bowl (return the husks to the bowl). Stir the bran mixture into the flour and cinnamon. Spoon into the prepared tin and smooth the surface. Bake for 45–50 minutes, or until cooked when a skewer inserted into the centre of the loaf comes out clean. Cool in the tin for 15 minutes, then turn out. Cut into thick slices to serve.

HINTS:
• Refrigerate in an airtight container for up to 5 days. You can freeze the loaf in individual slices wrapped in plastic wrap or foil for up to 1 month. Take out a slice for picnics or packed lunches.
• You can use any 2–3 varieties of dried fruit in this recipe, such as apricots, raisins, sultanas (golden raisins) or dates.

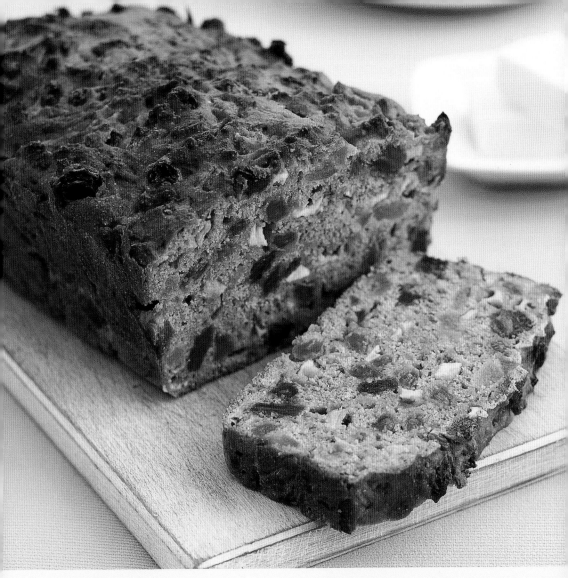

THIS WHOLESOME FRUIT LOAF
IS HIGH IN FIBRE, LOW IN FAT
AND MAKES A DELICIOUS
SNACK. YOU CAN ALSO ENJOY
IT FOR BREAKFAST OR BRUNCH,
EITHER FRESH OR TOASTED.

nutrition per slice: Energy 1057 kJ (252 Cal)

Fat 1 g

Saturated fat 0.2 g

Protein 6.5 g

Carbohydrate 51.6 g

Fibre 7.5 g

Cholesterol 1 mg

WINTER FRUIT IN ORANGE GINGER SYRUP

Sweet and nutritious, this fruity dessert is a good source of fibre and antioxidants. It's quite rich, so only a small amount of fruit is needed for each serve.

60 g (2¼ oz/¼ cup) caster (superfine) sugar
3 tbsp orange juice
2 strips orange peel
1 cinnamon stick
250 g (9 oz) dried fruit salad, large pieces cut in half

100 g (3½ oz) stoned dates
1 tsp grated fresh ginger
200 g (7 oz) low-fat plain yoghurt

Prep time: 10 minutes
Cooking time: 10 minutes
Serves 4

Put the sugar, orange juice, orange peel, cinnamon stick and 375 ml (13 fl oz/1½ cups) water in a large saucepan. Stir over low heat until the sugar dissolves, then increase the heat and simmer, without stirring, for 5 minutes, or until the syrup has thickened slightly.

Add the dried fruit salad, dates and ginger and toss well. Cover and simmer over low heat for 5 minutes, or until the fruit has softened. Remove the pan from the heat and set aside, covered, for 5 minutes. Discard the orange peel and cinnamon stick. If serving cold, remove the fruit from the saucepan and set aside to cool.

Place the fruit in individual serving dishes, top with the yoghurt and drizzle a little of the syrup over the top. Serve immediately.

nutrition per serve: Energy 1380 kJ (330 Cal); Fat 0.4 g; Saturated fat <0.1 g; Protein 5.5 g; Carbohydrate 74.1 g; Fibre 7.4 g; Cholesterol 2 mg

BAKED FIG AND RAISIN APPLES

THIS FRUIT DESSERT MAKES A TASTY AND FIBRE-RICH END TO A MEAL. YOU CAN VARY THE FILLING TO INCLUDE CHOPPED WALNUTS OR CURRANTS.

4 large cooking apples

80 g (2¾ oz/⅓ cup firmly packed) soft brown sugar

1½ tbsp chopped raisins

2 dried figs, chopped

½ tsp ground cinnamon (optional)

20 g (¾ oz) unsalted butter

low-fat yoghurt or ricotta cream (see Hints), to serve

PREP TIME: 10 MINUTES

COOKING TIME: 40 MINUTES

SERVES 4

Preheat the oven to 220°C (425°F/Gas 7). Core the apples and score the skin around the middle, so the apples won't burst while they are baking.

Combine the sugar, raisins, figs and cinnamon, if using. Place each apple on a piece of heavy-duty foil and fill the cavity with the fruit filling. Spread a little butter over the top of each apple, then wrap the foil securely around the apples. Bake for about 40 minutes, or until cooked through. Serve with yoghurt or ricotta cream.

HINTS:
• These apples can also be baked on a covered barbecue.
• To make the ricotta cream, whip equal quantities of low-fat ricotta cheese and low-fat plain yoghurt together and sweeten slightly with soft brown sugar. You can use this as a dip for fresh fruits, as a creamy filling for pastries or in place of whipped cream.

nutrition per serve: Energy 1054 kJ (252 Cal); Fat 4.5 g; Saturated fat 2.8 g; Protein 1.2 g; Carbohydrate 51 g; Fibre 5.8 g; Cholesterol 13 mg

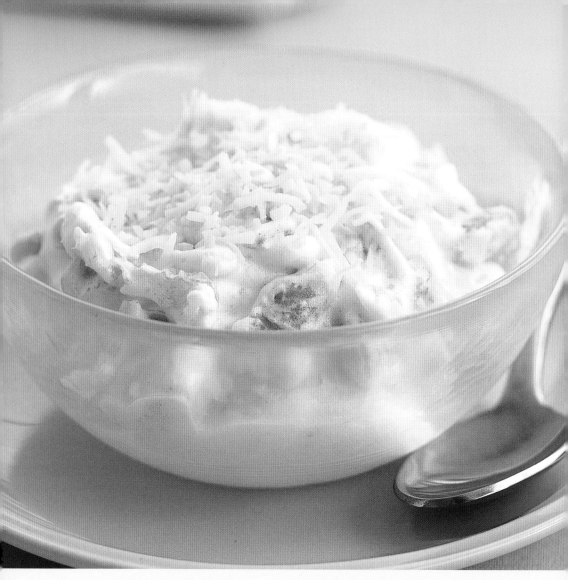

A FOOL IS A CLASSIC BRITISH
DESSERT TYPICALLY MADE WITH
PURÉED FRUIT AND WHIPPED
CREAM. THIS VERSION USES
EGG WHITES TO LIGHTEN THE
MIXTURE AND REDUCE THE FAT.
AND WE'VE ADDED SOME BRAN!

nutrition per serve: Energy 822 kJ (196 Cal)
Fat 2.1 g
Saturated fat 1.7 g
Protein 4.4 g
Carbohydrate 37.8 g
Fibre 5.9 g
Cholesterol 0 mg

DRIED APRICOT FOOL

30 g (1 oz) finely chopped glacé ginger
210 g (7½ oz) dried apricots, chopped
1 tbsp unprocessed wheat bran
2 egg whites
2 tbsp caster (superfine) sugar
2 tbsp shredded coconut, toasted

PREP TIME: 15 MINUTES
COOKING TIME: 5 MINUTES
SERVES 4

Place the ginger, apricots, wheat bran and 80 ml (2½ fl oz/⅓ cup) water in a small saucepan. Cook, covered, over very low heat for 5 minutes, stirring occasionally. Remove from the heat and allow to cool completely.

Using electric beaters, beat the egg whites in a clean, dry bowl until soft peaks form. Add the sugar and beat for 3 minutes, or until thick and glossy. Quickly and gently fold the cooled apricot mixture into the egg whites, and divide among four chilled serving glasses. Scatter the coconut over the top and serve immediately.

HINTS:
- The apricots can scorch easily, so cook over low heat.
- You need to serve this dessert immediately or the egg white will slowly break down and lose volume. If you want to do some earlier preparation, you can prepare the ginger and apricot mixture and leave in the refrigerator until needed.

Some websites with useful information

AUSTRALIA

Go Grains
http://gograins.grdc.com.au/index2.htm
Contains lots of information about the
health benefits of wholegrains.

The Cancer Council Australia
http://www.cancer.org.au

The Gut Foundation
www.gut.nsw.edu.au

Dietitians Association of Australia
http://www.daa.asn.au
At this site, you'll find healthy eating advice,
and you can also search for dietitians working
in your area.

The Healthy Eating Club
http://www.healthyeatingclub.org
Contains information about healthy
eating and nutrients.

GREAT BRITAIN

Cancer Research UK
http://www.cancerresearchuk.org

The British Dietetic Association
http://www.bda.uk.com

USA

National Digestive Diseases Information
Clearinghouse (NDDIC)
http://www.digestive.niddk.nih.gov
Has information on digestive diseases, such as
constipation, irritable bowel syndrome (IBS)
and diverticulosis.

National Cancer Institute
http://www.cancer.gov
This website contains lots of information about
various cancers, including colon cancer.

American Dietetic Association
www.eatright.org

OTHER USEFUL WEBSITES

Irritable Bowel Syndrome
Self Help and Support Group
http://www.ibsgroup.org

About Irritable Bowel Syndrome (IBS)
http://www.aboutibs.org

Glycemic Index (GI) and GI Database
www.glycemicindex.com

INDEX